And the
Silent Spoke

And the Silent Spoke

Amy L. Greeson

And the Silent Spoke

Copyright © 2019 by Amy L. Greeson
All rights reserved.

No part of this publication may be reproduced, stored in a retrieval system or transmitted in any way by any means, electronic, mechanical, photocopy, recording or otherwise without the prior permission of the author except as provided by USA copyright law.

The opinions expressed by the author are not necessarily those of Wisdom House Books, Inc.

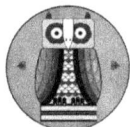

Published by Wisdom House Books, Inc.
Chapel Hill, North Carolina 27514 USA
1.919.883.4669 | www.wisdomhousebooks.com

Wisdom House Books is committed to excellence in the publishing industry.

Book design copyright © 2019 by Wisdom House Books, Inc. All rights reserved.

Cover and Interior Design by Ted Ruybal & Krystal Smith

Published in the United States of America

Paperback ISBN: 978-0-9994298-1-5
LCCN: 2019905974

BIO023000 | BIOGRAPHY & AUTOBIOGRAPHY / Adventurers & Explorers
MED040000 | MEDICAL / Holistic Medicine
TRV001000 | TRAVEL / Special Interest / Adventure

First Edition
14 13 12 11 10 / 10 9 8 7 6 5 4 3 2 1

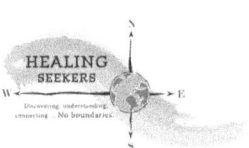

A percentage of the proceeds will be directed to the non-profit,

Healing Seekers
www.healingseekers.com
A 501c3 nonprofit educational organization.

I have tried to recreate events, locales and conversations from my memories of them. In order to maintain their anonymity in some instances I have changed the names of individuals and places, I may have changed some identifying characteristics and details such as physical properties, occupations and places of residence.

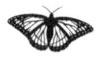
Dedication to

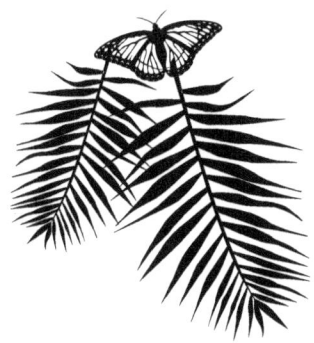

MM "Peggy" Reynolds—who has encouraged me to follow my passion and navigate this path in life while helping me to better understand the difficult points along the way. Thank you for expanding my world in so many ways, including through art and music, and for constantly reminding me to laugh. Thank you, most of all, for walking with me, and for your unbelievable love, patience and support during the months and years it took to write this book.

And to my parents, Joe and Barbara Greeson. If there really are angels on Earth, surely they are two of them. Thank you for encouraging me to live a life of love, to be compassionate to the struggles of others and to keep the faith.

A tremendous 'Thank You' to my publisher, Wisdom House Books—Ted Ruybal, Clara Jackson, Krystal Smith and Kelsey Campolong—for guiding me through this unknown territory. A special thank you to Kelsey, for editing, advising and helping me to birth more life into my words. You are amazing!

A special thank you to Annie Galvin Teich for editing and guiding me during the book's early stages. Thank you for the lessons, suggestions and guidance. And, for your friendship.

I would like to express my appreciation to:

The Expedition, Production and Post-Production, and Research Teams (past and present): Esteban Barrera, Core Expeditions, Celine Cousteau, John James, Neil Johnson, Josh Jones, Cary Kanoy, Grace Kanoy, Ryan Marie Kelly, Lori Leveille, Sherrie McWhorter, McWhorter Concepts, Martina Moore, Jeff Firewalker Schmitt, Diane Stevio, Capkin van Alphen and Wil Weldon.

Healing Seekers Board of Directors (past and present): Lindsay Burkart, Linda Carlisle, Dan Deuterman, Dawn Deuterman, Dennis Franks, Nancy Franks, Diana Hartje, Ogi Overman, Rita Rice-Ledford, Linda Riffle, Heath Slane and Annie Teich.

Natural Discoveries Board of Directors and Members: Bailey Gimbel, Eric Hill, Heath Slane and Landon Slane.

And my gratitude to:

The Molly Millis-Young Donor Advised Fund, The Emily Millis-Hiatt Donor Advised Fund, Judy Carter and Susan Sluyter, and The John C. and Marsha Slane Fund for the many years of tremendous support ~ and to the entire Healing Seekers family of donors and supporters ~ for making the educational materials and the Congo expedition and documentary possible.

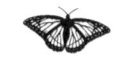
Table of Contents

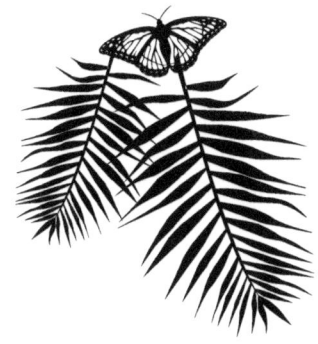

Chapter 1. 1

Chapter 2. 7

Chapter 3. 9

Chapter 4. 23

Chapter 5. 29

Chapter 6. 37

Chapter 7. 53

Chapter 8. 57

Chapter 9. 81

Chapter 10 95

Chapter 11 105

Chapter 12 107

Chapter 13 121

Chapter 14	127
Chapter 15	131
Chapter 16	145
Chapter 17	159
Chapter 18	167
Chapter 19	171
Chapter 20	187
Chapter 21	213
Chapter 22	221
Chapter 23	251
Chapter 24	257
Chapter 25	283
Chapter 26	295
Chapter 27	297
Chapter 28	323
Chapter 29	333
Chapter 30	339
Chapter 31	345
Chapter 32	347
Chapter 33	349
About the Author	353

Chapter One

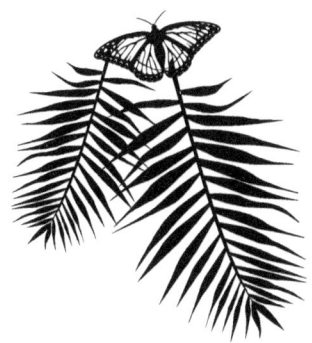

She held the small mirror and stared at its reflection. Her smooth youthful skin had long been replaced by deep lines and crevices. Her eyes, which had witnessed countless wonders, continued to fail . . . while her thick white hair waved ever so softly, proclaiming the elapsed years.

Slowly, she lifted her hand and gently wiped a tear that was forging a path across her cheek.

How can this be? How can this possibly be?

The changes to her physical appearance had taken decades, but to her they had come quickly. So quickly that she refused to claim the physical shell of the body as her own. This body had run marathons and triathlons and had trekked through some of the most pristine environments on Planet Earth. Yet there it was, fragile and worn by the years that had passed much too swiftly.

God, she prayed, please tell me that there was purpose and benefit for the days that I walked this Earth . . . that somehow, I made a difference . . . that somehow, my life was not in vain.

Spiritually, her heart was at peace. But there was also a heaviness. She had hoped to accomplish so much more in life, but no matter how hard she had tried, there remained incurable diseases, incomplete research, untapped destinations and unfulfilled time with loved ones.

Only in the latter years did she finally begin to realize that it had not been the countless days of work or the months exploring jungles and indigenous villages that were the most significant in life. And it had not been the accomplishments and successes that brought the greatest moments of joy. Rather, it had been the love, and the love freely shared, that had made life worthwhile. The relationships, connections . . . the chance encounters. These were the special moments of bonding in which the very fabric of life had been beautifully woven. Moments that had been divinely guided and orchestrated. And moments in which joy had often been so overwhelming that it had taken her breath away.

Foregoing retirement in her sixties, she continued to work into her early eighties, immersing herself in the research that had always invigorated her soul. Although she limited her travels, she continued to guide and coordinate many of the expeditions and plant collections.

Overall, her life seemed a blur, packed with daily activities through which she yearned to better understand the world and make a positive impact upon it, while also struggling with self-improvement. The drive to make a difference had been unrelenting and so intense that she had rarely left its embrace.

That was, until one day. Three years earlier.

A mid-morning phone call at the laboratory had sent her rushing to the hospital. Within an hour of her arrival, her life partner died in her arms. They had spent forty years together and other than the expeditions, had rarely been apart.

The depth of heartbreak was incomprehensible. The sudden loss

Chapter One

unbearable. And the agony beyond description. So devastating was the implosion in her heart that she too wanted to die.

Instead, she completely withdrew from society and retreated to their simple home located in the midst of a hundred acres of pristine forest. Its isolation and silence cradled her, bringing moments of great peace. And yet, interspersed were endless days in which she felt hopelessly lonely.

The alienation from society quickly transformed her formerly robust, outgoing persona into a quiet, withdrawn, introverted one. Days were often spent berating herself over the time that she and her love had been apart; days in which she had chosen to spend months on expeditions and with research. Time which she could not retrieve and moments which she could not erase and re-do.

Conversations beyond her immediate family became practically nonexistent. It was as if she lived in her own virtual monastery.

Yet, it was in this hermitage that she began to relive much of her life . . . and its many chapters. Each chapter had its own conglomeration of experiences, interactions, and personal discoveries that formed the essence of who she had become. The trials and tribulations along the way had also created her and forever impacted the way she envisioned the world and the work that had become her life's mission.

Throughout the years she had shared many of these stories of her life, but the depth and intensity of them had only been shared with one person. Her life partner. Their conversations had been deep, intimate and shared within a space so safe that she spontaneously bared her innermost feelings and divulged her most private thoughts. But her life partner, the confidant who had always been there, was no longer with her. And the moments that had once belonged to two were now fragmented and coveted only by one.

The more she thought of these stories and moments in her life, the greater the urge to share them. The desire to do so came not from a place of ego or from selfish desire; rather, it surfaced from a desire to help others in *their journeys of life. Those others whom she longed to help and to guide were her nieces and nephews.*

The best aunt she was not, but there had always been a special place in her heart for each of her nieces and nephews. She had watched them grow, taking immense pride in the individuals they had become. And it was because of her love for them that almost three years to the day, she emerged from the seclusion, ended the silence and opened her heart once more.

Boldly, she had sent each of them an airline ticket requesting that they join her the following month for a three-day weekend. She was thrilled that each had accepted, including the two who lived in Alaska. She imagined the stories she would hear about their families, careers and lives. And she also fantasized about the things she would share.

She hoped that her words would help pilot them. And perhaps make their paths a bit easier.

The month since sending the invitations passed quickly, and soon the house would come alive once more. For on the following day, they were slated to arrive.

Now, though, it was time for bed, and she needed to rest. Her health had plummeted in the past two years. Two light strokes and a severely weakened heart had taken its toll, causing her body to become weak and frail.

Even holding the mirror became a struggle, as her arm weakened and fell to her side. Unable to continue its hold, her hand released its grip, sending the mirror on a collision course with the hardwood floor below.

Sighing deeply, she closed her eyes.

Chapter One

With labored breaths, she knew it would not be long before her body could no longer sustain the life that now flowed through it. Quietly, she vowed to be strong, determined to enjoy every minute with her nieces and nephews and to say the things left unsaid.

Over the next three days, she would share with them what had become her most cherished and valuable treasures: the experiences and lessons of a lifetime and the love that had become her.

During those days, her soul would soar, and her heart would burst with joy.

And it was during that time that the years of solitude and isolation broke . . .

And the silent one spoke

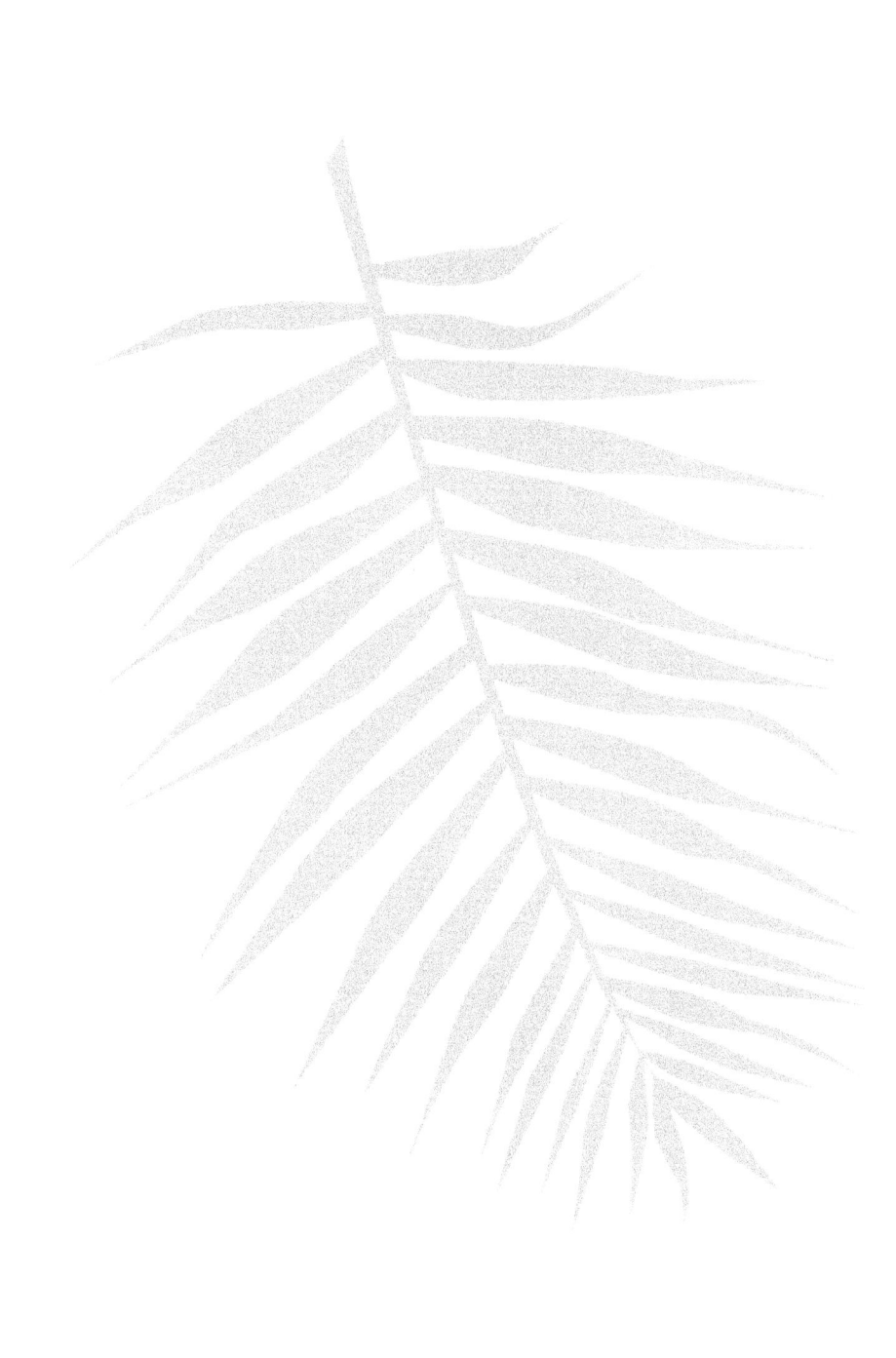

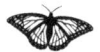

Chapter Two

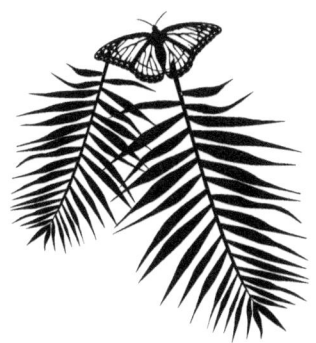

It had been eleven years since all the nieces and nephews had gathered in one place. The first two kids arrived near noon and the others shortly thereafter. Each gently hugging and greeting her with a kiss.

For a while, all she could do was smile and listen to their voices.

Every meal for the weekend had been carefully planned, created by Dominga, her caretaker and friend. The house had also been immaculately cleaned; the finest linens and sheets had been set out and every conceivable amenity was made available.

While the kids talked, Dominga placed large trays of fresh rolls, chicken and shrimp skewers, and bowls of curried vegetables for them to enjoy. There were also platters of fresh fruit and homemade cookies along with a selection of beverages, including a large pitcher of sweet tea.

With multiple conversations taking place simultaneously, the nieces and nephews mingled freely, speaking to one and then another. Conversations included travel and sports, job situations and graduations, and remembrances of childhood. For a couple of hours, they reminisced. And she, with them. It had been three years since such love and happiness had filled the home. And her heart.

Although there was much joy, there was also sadness as conversations shifted to loved ones who had passed and to a family member whose health had recently taken a sudden turn for the worse.

Wishing to comfort them and not wanting there to be further sadness, she softly cleared her throat and began to speak.

Life is a spectacular adventure. If you're lucky, the times of joy far surpass those of sadness. No matter the situation, if you are surrounded with love, as you are now, you will be the luckiest of all.

For all the things I have witnessed and experienced in my life . . . I wish for you so much more.

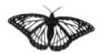

Chapter Three

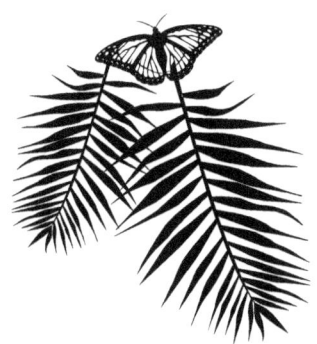

S*canning the room, she paused briefly at each niece and nephew, looking at each face to give a moment's undivided attention before continuing.*

Some of you know exactly what you want in life. The rest of you, like me, may need years to figure it out.

It wasn't until I was almost thirty years old that I truly began to grasp who I was, my path and purpose in life. When I began exploring the world's jungles with their degrees of complexity, I began to further explore the world within myself. Each journey became a teacher . . . and the experiences often led to epiphanies and revelations.

It was my third trip to the Amazon. This one into a stunning region of Peru. As with the two prior trips, the Amazon seemed to beckon me. My heart pounded with excitement and my eyes beheld what I believed to be one of the most beautiful and lush places on Planet Earth.

The Amazon summoned the free spirit, the introvert, the explorer and the spiritual seeker. It delicately embraced every life form and yet simultaneously wove each organism into its complicated matrix.

Travel to our destination required six to seven hours along the Amazon River and another three and a half hours traveling one of its tributaries. The trip began before sunrise and was only interrupted by two brief stops along the river's banks. It was hot, humid, and the jungle was throbbing with the intensity of life.

Our group of seven came from different regions: California, Wisconsin, Oregon, Hawaii, Barcelona, and North Carolina. Leading the trip was Andie, a good friend of mine who was at the forefront of natural medicine. For years she had been apprenticing with Miguel, an Amazonian medicine man, also known as a shaman. Our trip was the first time Miguel was permitting any outsiders to join them.

Base camp was located fifty yards from the tributary's eastern bank. The site allowed easy access for land or water exploration, day or night. Boarding a small boat in the morning on the second day, we traveled upstream with Miguel and our boat driver and guide, Carlos.

The boat, engulfed by dense jungle on either side, chugged slowly along the waterway's narrow, winding path as Carlos weaved back and forth, dodging clumps of floating vegetation. The vegetation was known locally as river lettuce, and it could easily become entangled in the outboard motor. Its bright green color was in stark contrast to the tributary's black water, which was the result of abundant tannins from the jungle's decomposing trees and vegetation.

From the dark waters, pink dolphins surfaced only to re-submerge around and under the boat. Known as botos, the Amazon

Chapter Three

river dolphins are thought to be the largest river dolphins in the world. The young are primarily gray, but with maturity they develop the characteristic pink color. Especially the males.

Although it appeared as if they had come to play, the dolphins were likely feasting on the piranhas, croakers and other species of fish, which had been disoriented by the churning of water caused by our small outboard motor. And even though the tributary's black, murky water prevented much visibility, it was no deterrent to their mastery of echolocation in finding their prey.

The larger tributary on which we traveled was fed by numerous smaller ones. Veering off onto one of them, Carlos followed a tapering path of twists and turn which dwindled until it was only ten feet wide. Tree limbs, branches and vegetation brushed against us as we ducked and pushed them aside, trying to avoid cuts and scrapes. Foremost in my mind however, were thoughts of possible stinging and biting insects and venomous snakes which might be knocked off of the limbs into the boat or onto one of us.

The narrow waterway eventually led into a stagnant, swampy lake. Trees protruded sporadically from the lake's shallow water while giant water lilies floated on the surface. The water lilies were enormous. Known as *Victoria amazonica*, they were round and flat with upraised edges, resulting in diameters of up to six and eight feet. Carlos explained that the larger ones could support a weight of seventy to eighty pounds. Or more.

Emerging from the lilies' bright green circular bases were spectacular white, pink and purple flowers, which dotted the distant landscape like large balls of cotton. Whiffs of their fruity sweetness filled the air and mingled with the jungle's woodsy, earthy aroma.

After a couple of hours, Carlos turned the boat around to go back toward the main tributary. As he did so, sudden loud, intense squawking and groaning noises pulled our attention upwards into the tree canopy.

Thirty feet above, a hoatzin perched on a limb. Its crest was wildly spiked and its face, bright blue. With reddish-brown eyes, he peered down upon us as he expanded and contracted his wings while turning around in small circles.

Also known as reptile birds, the hoatzins are born with claws underneath their wings. If a young one falls from the nest, the claws are used to climb the tree in order to return to the nest. The species seemed to be a classic example of natural selection from Darwin's book, *On the Origin of Species.*

Parrots and macaws, squirrel monkeys, capuchins and howler monkeys kept us company as we made our way back to the larger tributary, turned right, and headed further upstream. At some point, Miguel motioned for Carlos to steer the boat toward a particular tree. The tree was large with wide branches that reached close to the water's edge. From a distance, it looked much like an old oak tree. The leaves, Miguel explained, were used in a preparation to treat diarrhea.

Although the treatment was intriguing, I was more interested in the reprieve of the tree's shade. It was exceptionally hot and the air heavy, and I was saturated in sweat.

As I relaxed and enjoyed the relief from the sun, there was a sudden sharp inflection in Miguel's voice, which brought my full attention back to him. As our guide translated his words, Miguel asked if anyone could see the snake that was within six feet of us. We all looked, straining to see the creature we knew was there. My eyes began to squint as if somehow it would help me to see more clearly. I looked closely at the roots of the tree near the water's edge, along the trunk and its limbs and across the water itself. I peered into the nearby foliage but saw nothing.

Chapter Three

For ten minutes we all searched, but not one person in our group of outdoor enthusiasts could see the snake. Not one.

Then, Miguel stood, and with the end of a paddle, pointed above our heads. We still could not see it. Extending his arm, he used the paddle to gently touch the snake before separating it from the tree and bringing the snake closer for us to see. A green vine snake. It was an extension of the limb itself—almost impossible to distinguish where the tree limb ended and the snake began. I cringed, realizing how disconnected and unaware the seven of us medical professionals were in this environment.

Life is often like that. Sometimes things appear right before our eyes and yet we're unable to see them. Sometimes it's only because of another that our eyes are opened and our perspective shifts. And with the shift, the world is seen in an entirely new light.

With each passing day, I became more immersed in the jungle's rhythm and flow. Even though there were millions of life forms and hundreds of sounds, there existed stillness. And even with the tremendous numbers of insects, microbes, plants and animals, there existed individuality. Single organisms thrived and at the same time merged with other life forms to create a body of life that seemed infinite. And with the infinity was an endless serenity.

The days were passing quickly, and there was not enough time to see and absorb even a fraction of the Amazon's wonders. Yet, as daylight faded, the evenings brought forth other worlds to explore.

At night, the jungle sings a wonderful lullaby. It is like a combination of stringed instruments and percussionists performing a symphony of staccatos and legatos, of tenors and sopranos. I could rarely guess the voice, the musician, or the size of the orchestra.

And it didn't matter.

Every night there was a different performance, and as I stretched out underneath my mosquito net, I listened until I drifted off to sleep.

Day seven began like any other day. I awoke before daylight with a multitude of life forms: insects, birds, and monkeys. The mornings began softly, and with every passing minute, the volume would go up a decibel as a few more members joined the jungle's chorus. Most mornings, with the sound of macaws close by, I would quickly slide from underneath my mosquito net to catch a glimpse as they flew overhead.

The jungle was as magical on the seventh day as it had been on the first. After a breakfast of granola and fruit, I prepared for the day of hiking. Placing my camera into a small waterproof bag, I placed it inside my backpack before stuffing in a bottle of water and a bag of trail mix. Strapping the pack on my back, I joined with the others in forming a single line behind Miguel.

I hiked with eyes wide open . . . fascinated by the variety of butterflies, including the blue morphos. With wings of iridescent blue rimmed in black, the blue morphos' wing spans were often five to eight inches. They looked more like small birds except that they flittered through the forest following a trajectory that appeared both spastic and sporadic.

Chapter Three

Dragonflies, mosquitoes and other flying insects darted all around us, dodging the plants and trees as well as the numerous cobwebs. We, on the other hand, seemed to keep running into the webs, collecting their silky strands across our faces, arms and torsos.

Common were spectacular flowers like the *Heliconia*, which is also known as lobster-claw because of the striking resemblance to a lobster's red claws. The jungle's flora seemed to overlap and weave together, giving the appearance of one endless species of life, occupying every square inch of soil.

Like a child bursting with anticipation with every twist and turn of the path and with every strike of the shaman's machete, I was on a roller coaster ride of endorphins. Periodically Miguel would stop, point to something, pick it up or chop it off and tell us all about it. There were plants, barks, roots, and berries that were used locally for infection and inflammation, for worms, vomiting and malaria. There were saps and leaves used for pregnancy, pain and coughing.

I imagined a child with horrific vomiting and diarrhea. A man with a broken leg. And a woman hemorrhaging from childbirth. There were no IVs, no medical clinics, no x-rays or CT scans, no sanitary conditions, much less clean water.

I thought about Western medicine and its arsenal of treatments, devices and equipment. I thought of how I had taken such things for granted and felt sad that the advances in western medicine were not available to everyone. And then I remembered that a great percentage of the world's population relied solely on nature and community healers for treatments with an astonishing rate of success. Nature was and had always been the alpha laboratory, and those who lived within it were keepers of priceless wisdom and knowledge. In more ways than I had ever imagined.

I thought of my father back home, holding down the family pharmacy. In pharmacy school, he had been taught pharmacognosy, the study of medications derived from plants and natural resources. I, however, had not. No one—no professor, drug representative—no commercial, advertisement—not one source had ever explained the full degree to which natural resources had been the blueprints to more than half of our pharmaceuticals.

These products that had been patterned or derived from nature were pharmaceuticals that I dispensed hundreds of times a week. They included antibiotics, diabetic medications, chemo drugs, heart medicines, blood pressure medications and blood thinners. And it was often due to the information that was shared by an indigenous person or healer that such discoveries were made possible.

I was glimpsing a profound truth: the world was more dependent upon these indigenous healers and their environments than the indigenous people and environments were dependent upon Westerners. Little did I know at that moment how this insight would alter the course of my life.

The sounds of the jungle changed with every passing hour. And with them, my thoughts. To be a part of something so grand, even momentarily, is humbling.

As I hiked, I melted into its rhythm of life. I was impressed with Miguel's knowledge of plants and remedies, yet, it would later be the spiritual component that captivated me the most.

We returned to camp several hours later in the afternoon, tired and hungry. We reeked of insect repellent and sweat, a smell to which we had become accustomed. Dips in the river and rinsing

Chapter Three

off in a makeshift shower were welcomed treats, even though the cleanliness was temporary.

Before grabbing a late lunch, several of us chatted briefly about the morning's trek. As we stood and talked, we swatted at the barrage of insects—a never-ending arsenal of mosquitoes, flies and other unknown creatures—which found our sweaty DEET bodies appealing. The swatting motion had become second nature since our arrival, slapping and waving almost unconsciously at anything that made contact with us. It was one thing to keep them off of you because they were annoying, but quite another to prevent bites, which could cause an unknown number of reactions and problems.

As we talked, I became more and more irritated at the creature that would not leave the back of my right leg alone. While talking and maintaining eye contact with my friends, I kept swatting without success. Finally, I slapped the back of my leg with intense force, determined to get rid of the insect for good.

It was a moment that I would quickly regret.

Immediately, I felt penetrating jabs into the crevices of the third and fourth fingers of my right hand. The stings were painful and felt as if seven or eight hornets had simultaneously stung the same two centimeters, right in the delicate folds of my tender flesh. While saying a few choice words, I turned around to look at my calf. Tears formed in my eyes while I strained to see the culprit. Raising my leg slightly, I stared as if in a momentary daze. There, stuck to the back of my leg, was a spiny caterpillar.

Its spines protruded outward like erect porcupine quills. My skin was no match for its protective armor. Carlos squatted and peered intently at the creature on my leg, then stood up and left. He returned a few minutes later with a piece of bark with which to pry it off.

Afterwards, I could not quit thinking about the incident, and it bothered me well into the evening. Even though there had been no pain beyond the initial penetrations, no stinging, itching, redness, irritation or inflammation, there was the disturbing, lingering thought that a creature had crawled up my leg and attached itself to my body without my immediate awareness. How long had it been there? What other insects, parasites, etcetera might be on my body of which I was also unaware?

It was from that point on that I became preoccupied with visually inspecting every inch of my body . . . and I mean every inch of my body, every evening. And though the others never admitted to it, I am certain that they did the same.

Days passed and other stories took precedent over the rehashing of my caterpillar companion. When our group returned to camp late one night, I decided to head to the makeshift shower for a quick rinse before joining the others for a bite to eat. Even though my headlamp provided several feet of light directly in front of me, darkness persisted above, behind and to either side. Never far from my mind were thoughts of jaguars, as Carlos had discovered fresh tracks through camp the first morning after our arrival.

The shower was simple: a single small tube funneled the water from the nearest tributary and a valve controlled its slow flow. The surrounding four walls were composed of wooden slabs with small spaces in between. Only four feet by four and a half feet in size, the area was small but afforded a level of privacy.

I eagerly looked forward to the soap and water cleanse followed by clean, dry clothes. Positioning the headlamp just right on the ground allowed the light to be directed to the shower valve, while also providing several feet of dim light. I tossed my soiled clothes in the corner away from the water and reached for my bottle of biodegradable soap. It was a great feeling to have the

Chapter Three

water gently move over my neck and down my back. Thoughts of the day's adventures flooded my mind as I washed my hair and then lathered the rest of my body. Bathing became pretty much unconscious, as every thought was about the jungle and the things I had seen and experienced that day.

Suddenly though, the smooth up and down motion of my soapy hands washing my right leg came to an abrupt halt as the ends of my fingers came in contact with something that was wrapped around my ankle. The discovery caused a shock to go through my body.

From the brief contact, I knew that it was lumpy and bulbous... and yet soft. Whatever it was, it had a tight grip on my right ankle and wasn't letting go. How could I have not seen this earlier? I had been wearing shorts with my Teva river sandals, so it wasn't like my ankles had been covered by socks and boots. How did I not feel this on my body? How could someone else not have noticed?

I began to panic.

In all my outdoor experiences, I had never had a creature attach itself to me, and this was the second time in just a few days.

I knew that I needed to find Carlos in the event it was harmful or poisonous, so that he could once again remove a creature from my body. Tip-toeing like I had an injured right foot, I hobbled a few steps to grab my headlamp and my glasses, and then reluctantly aimed the light toward the ankle.

Part of me didn't want to look. And part of me couldn't wait to know. I aimed the light on the spot and slowly bent down to get a closer look. I stood motionless and could not believe my eyes.

There, wrapped all the way around my ankle, was not a poisonous creature or anything deadly or harmful... or even alive. There, tightly bound, was the handcrafted anklet that in my wandering mind I had forgotten all about. Earlier in the day a young woman from a local tribe had gifted it to me, placing it around my ankle.

I didn't know whether to laugh or cry. I think I did both.

I quickly finished my shower and joined the others. As I told the story, they laughed until they cried.

That night, I thought at length about what had happened. I was relieved and yet, my fear both surprised and concerned me.

The angst I had in the shower would likely have never happened had it not been for the incident with the spiny caterpillar a few days earlier. The caterpillar had instilled a level of fear and defensiveness toward the jungle and its creatures that didn't exist prior to that point in time, causing a shift that resulted in heightened apprehension. And it unsettled me.

I didn't want to live my life based on fear, anxiety, panic and dread. I wanted to return to the 'me' that didn't overreact and was not afraid.

Sometimes in the blink of an eye, something happens, and we change. If we're lucky, though, things are brought to our awareness and we learn valuable lessons.

I wondered how many 'caterpillars' had unknowingly affected my life and were still holding on. How many times had I responded inappropriately, avoided something or prematurely judged something or someone based on an event, misconception or misguided thought?

I vowed to be more attentive. I prayed for fear to no longer have a hold on me. And I prayed even more for God to spare me any more surprises on the trip . . . real or imagined.

When I began to understand that many of my fears were simply imagined, I felt empowered. It was me who had birthed, fed and nurtured them. And it was me who had the power to cut their lifelines.

Chapter Three

Like the previous two trips, I became sad when it was time to leave the jungle. The jungle's world was vastly different than that from which I came. Within it existed a serenity and peace in which joy and survival were dependent upon living in the present moment.

Each day in the jungle I felt as if I had returned to a childlike state in which I ceaselessly marveled at its wonders and beauty, with inextinguishable eagerness and excitement. Leaving its embrace felt as if I was leaving a part of my soul behind.

I had gone into the jungle to learn its healing powers and for the adventure. I emerged realizing that the greatest experience and adventure had been that which had taken place within myself.

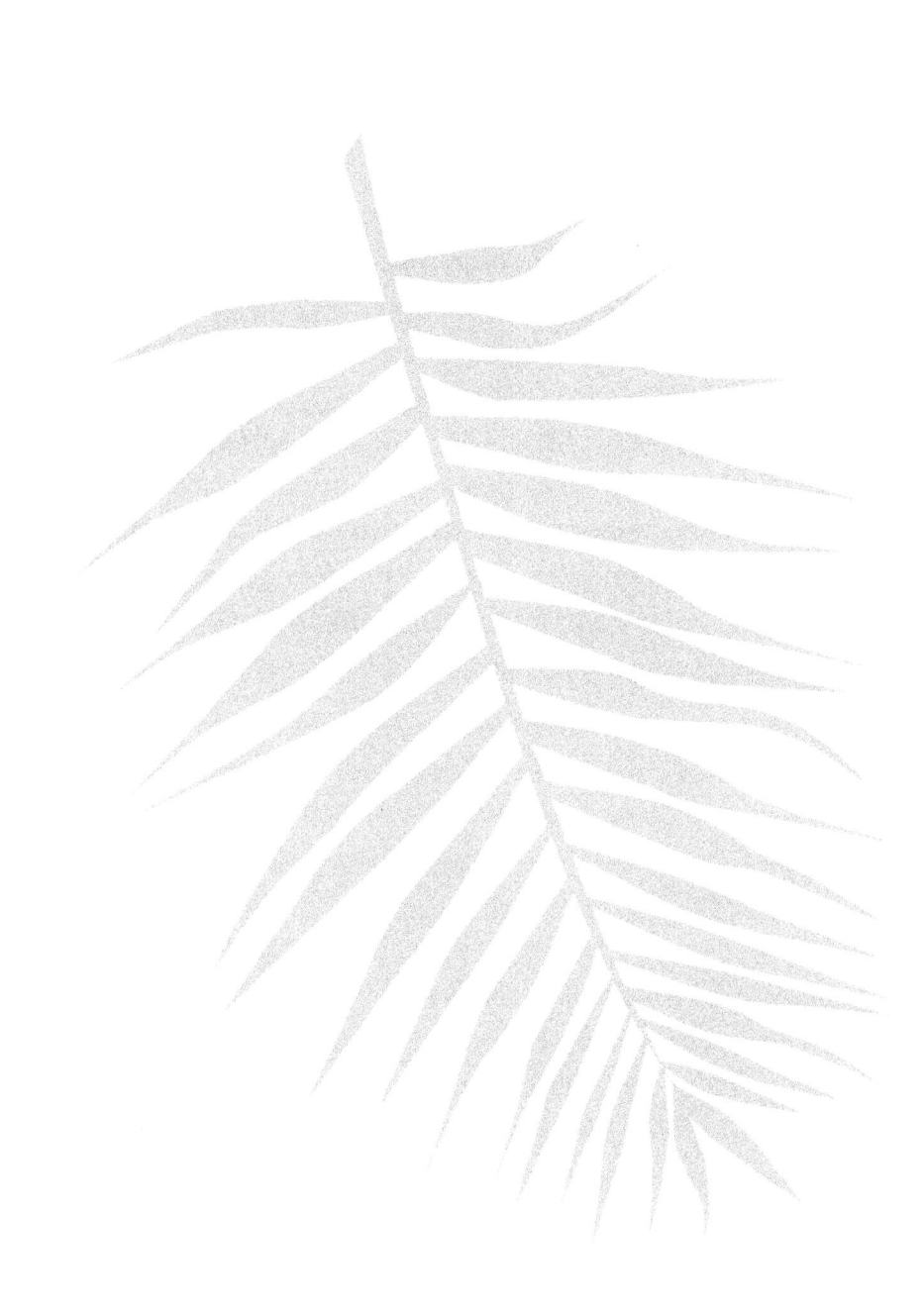

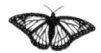

Chapter Four

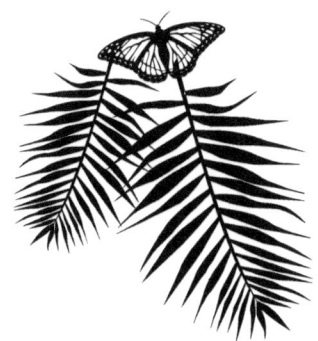

Returning back home to North Carolina, my normal routine resumed. Instead of days trekking through the jungle, days were spent working at the pharmacy, gathering with friends and family, cycling, kayaking and reading.

While in Barnes & Noble one day searching for a new book, I was immediately intrigued by a new release. Thumbing through the pages of the book, the chapters described several animals, insects and creatures whose chemical compounds were used to defend themselves against predators. Such chemicals, ironically, have also led to the development of pharmaceuticals.

After purchasing the book, I went straight home, stretched out across the sofa and began to read. Flipping through the pages, I came across one particular insect that I recognized all too well. The book's photo of a small porcupine-like organism seemed to be the same spiny caterpillar that had hitchhiked on the back of my leg just three months earlier. After reading the information about the genus *Lonomia*, I closed the book and looked at its cover once more.

And the Silent Spoke

The book was a compilation of some of nature's most dangerous and venomous creatures. The entry stated that the caterpillar's poisonous compounds could cause delayed cerebral and abdominal hemorrhaging. Even though I rarely damage a book, I didn't think twice about ripping out the two pages in order to fax them over to my doctor the following morning. At the top of the first page, I wrote a short note describing the incident in the jungle and asked for his advice.

Within thirty minutes the doctor's nurse called, recommending that several tests be done as soon as possible. The next day I went to the hospital for blood work and scans.

In the hours that followed as I waited for the results, my thoughts and fears escalated. Was I bleeding in the brain and abdomen? It had been three months since the incident. Was there already permanent damage, too late for treatment? Had I made a huge mistake by going to the jungle?

A day later, a phone call with a cheerful hello from the nurse immediately put me at ease. The results were fine. No abnormalities were detected. Blood work and scans were great.

It was at that point that I told my parents the whole story, sharing the book's information about the toxins found in the caterpillar's stinging spines. To tell them before I knew all the details would have caused them to worry incessantly. But worry they did, even after the good news, knowing that I had dreams of traveling to other jungles. Jungles where many other poisonous and deadly creatures existed.

Several days later while we were both working at the pharmacy, my father took me aside and delicately, said, "On your next trip why don't you go somewhere like Austria or Germany? It's beautiful there and you've never been to Europe." His message

Chapter Four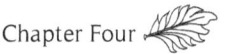

was clear. He was afraid that an incident, like with the caterpillar, would happen again . . . and perhaps with a worse outcome. His words were loving, and I must admit that a part of me was happy to hear them, as I too had become somewhat fearful of the jungle and its creatures.

Ironically, the following year, I was invited to go to Europe with my great friend, Marie. Although Scotland and London sounded like wonderful places to visit, they had never been at the top of my bucket list. I was, however, looking forward to the time with my friend and excited to be going somewhere that was safer than a jungle.

It was our third day in London and the date was July 5th, 2005. The day began like any other day but ended like no other. For on that day, terrorist suicide bombers attacked London.

While strolling around the city, Marie and I had stopped at an outside market to shop. Moments later, there was a loud explosive blast with a force so intense it felt like the pavement itself was shaking. For a few moments, we were motionless as the city stood still. And then, the city's paralysis broke into an awkward commotion.

We walked closer to a merchant's stand where several others had migrated, all straining to hear a small radio. There was little information, only that there had been two or more bombs . . . and something about a bus. And a backpack. As we listened, sirens filled the air. Emergency vehicles, police, fire.

Around the merchant's stand, Marie and I stood shoulder to shoulder with other locals and tourists who were of various nationalities, cultures, races, and ages. Empathy, concern and kindness overflowed. Questions streamed, as we asked one another if he or she was okay, where they lived or where they were staying, how they were getting home, and if they needed anything.

In that moment, there was an overwhelming sense of unity. In that moment, it was as if everyone gathered around the merchant's stand was family.

No one, however, took charge. No one knew what to do. Gradually, the group dispersed. Marie and I, too, departed to make our way back to the only place we felt we would be safe. Our hotel.

As we nervously walked, questions came quickly one after another in my mind. Was there a bomb in the bus that was passing? What about the taxi cab? Or the people carrying backpacks we were getting ready to walk by? Was it safer to walk on this side of the street or on that side? Would we be better off to just stay where we were?

There was no direction, no instruction. There were no answers. There was no reassurance or any feeling of safety.

Many people wanted to leave London as soon as possible. Airlines reported that all available seats on departing flights had been quickly filled. For all those who remained in London, however, there was nothing to do but hope and pray that the attacks were over.

Our scheduled flight back to the U.S.A. was still two days out. Although we debated leaving London immediately and going to France, we realized that France, too, might be a target for atrocious acts of violence. So, we remained for two more days in London.

People seem to come together in a crisis. There is kindness and comfort from strangers, regardless of ethnicity, social, or economic status. The heightened empathy toward others demonstrates love on the highest level. And that level of love is the epitome of altruism.

On that day, complete strangers found comfort in one another. Human kindness transcended into bonds of love, and in the midst of great angst, I glimpsed the potential of humanity.

Chapter Four

Many times in my life I have been frightened and even terrified. Moments in which I felt powerless and helpless, even though the moments were often sudden and fleeting. Being charged by a grizzly bear, being near three avalanches, in the blinding ash of a volcanic eruption, in numerous earthquakes, being arrested twice in a foreign country, within a few feet of a *fer-de-lance*, etcetera. But those experiences paled in comparison to the terror I felt in London that day and the two days that followed.

It was a fear that surpassed any of my harrowing experiences in nature or in any remote area of the world. There was nothing . . . nothing . . . nothing more horrifying than the evil intentions of a human being.

On our flight back to the United States two days later, I became emotional as I realized that millions of people live in war-torn areas and face such conflicts on a daily basis. I could not fully comprehend what that entailed. I imagined it to be living in constant fear, struggling every day for survival, and helplessly trying to protect a family. How does one survive? Much less thrive? They were people just like me, people with family and friends. They were good people who just happened to be in horrific situations.

For those few days in London I had insight into such a life, and I realized that when tragedy strikes, love can embrace us in the most powerful and unexpected ways. During that time, the unity of humanity was cultivated and it prevailed, and it was not for a moment powerless to any terrorist activity or evil. Humanity was not separated by barriers based on race, religion or belief.

I breathed a sigh of relief, grateful for our safety. And yet a disturbing truth lingered. Unlike Marie and me, millions of people in the world had no escape and had to live without freedom and safety.

My heart sank as the sadness overwhelmed me. Before this incident, I had not felt such a level of empathy for people in war-torn areas. I had never imagined their circumstances or difficulties, and I was ashamed that my heart had been so disconnected.

When you walk in another's shoes, you begin to awaken to their world. And you also awaken a part of yourself that has perhaps remained dormant until that very moment.

It became clear to me that it was not through human eyes that I was seeing the world, but through the eyes of the divine heart. It was through these eyes that I could see the reflections of my own soul, the interconnections of all life, and the bonds of love which embrace us all.

This cascade of events in my life had originated with a caterpillar. A creature whose metamorphosis transforms its gravity-bound larva into a free-flying butterfly . . . one of the most beautiful and peaceful life forms on Earth.

I slowly began to see the transformations taking place within myself.

And I faintly began to see the metamorphosis of my own life.

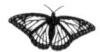

Chapter Five

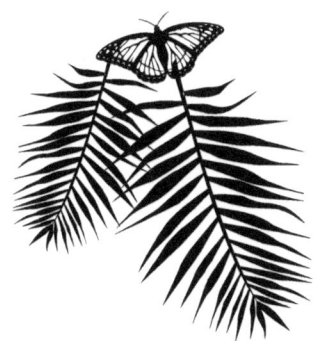

Life was unfolding in ways and dimensions that I had never imagined. The world and its life forms were far more complex and expansive than I had ever fathomed, and as my mind expanded, so did the dreams of discovering new treatments and cures.

In my role as a pharmacist, I also spent countless hours consulting customers and patients on the safe use of herbals, botanicals and nutraceuticals, often in combination with prescription medications. Natural medicine was new territory for most people in our small conservative town, and as a medical professional, I had to tread lightly.

I quickly gained a reputation as a natural medicine pharmacist and furthered my studies in every way possible. This included attending conferences across the country and earning the only certification available at the time for a pharmacist specializing in integrative medicine.

Every person with whom I worked was unique, and each had his or her own thoughts as to what was the right 'medicine' for him or her. For some, it was only pharmaceuticals, while others added a limited range of vitamins. Still others sought regimens of only herbal, botanical and alternative therapies. However, the majority of people with whom I worked sought a blend of both the natural and the pharmaceutical.

Many of them were desperate for cures and came to me as a last resort. With a heavy heart, I listened as they tearfully explained their diagnoses, the unsuccessful treatments and the doctor's final words . . . that Western medicine had no solutions for the issues they faced. Some were given months to live, others just weeks, while still others were simply told they would experience an eventual slow demise.

Although the integrative medicine consulting was challenging, I enjoyed being of service in this way. It inspired me to learn more about herbal and pharmaceutical treatments as well as the conditions and diseases that patients were tackling. The dietary supplements, herbal products and pharmaceuticals were often very beneficial, but I dreamed of the day when treatments would be discovered that would cure once and for all.

More times than I care to remember, I dispensed prescriptions and took care of patients who heroically fought illnesses and diseases only to eventually lose their battles. Some of these warriors I'd known much of my life—or most of their lives. They were friends and friends' parents, grandparents, siblings, spouses and children. They were teachers and factory workers, realtors and coaches, doctors and nurses, ministers and some of the greatest kickball players and winners of hide-and-seek.

As their diseases progressed and their conditions worsened, patients required stronger medications and more elaborate treatment regimens. I watched them weaken to the point that they could

Chapter Five

no longer walk and talk, communicate or respond. I watched as their family members and friends suffered emotionally and struggled daily, bearing a weight that no one should ever have to bear.

And with great sadness, I read their obituaries and listened to their eulogies.

I was tired of the sadness. I was exhausted by my feelings of helplessness. And so, perhaps for no other reason than to feel like I was doing something, I decided that I would try to find the cures myself.

It was 2008, the year that marked the first expedition in which I would actively pursue new treatments. Previous trips had been incredible learning experiences, but they did not involve the actual collection of plants for analysis and study.

To find treatments that had not already been studied by other researchers in the world, I had to go to some of the more isolated and remote areas of the planet; places where there were higher probabilities of novel species and compounds as yet undiscovered by Western science. Places where there was little to no documentation of scientific study. At the top of the list was Madagascar.

Madagascar is known as one of the most highly bio-diverse lands in the world. The abundance and variety of life that exist on the small island include thousands of species thought to exist nowhere else on the planet.

Gravely, it is also considered one of the areas most threatened with habitat loss.

One species that calls Madagascar home is *Catharanthus roseus*, better known as the rosy periwinkle. With five soft, rose-colored petals that gently overlap one another, the flower has been used by generations of the Malagasy people for treating health conditions, including high blood sugar. Like many plants in their natural habitats, the rosy periwinkle has developed chemical compounds that it uses to defend and protect itself. Unable to run away when it is threatened by a predator or other danger, the plant secretes these chemical arsenals to harm or kill whatever is threatening it. Typically, insects or microbes.

In the 1950's, scientists studying the rosy periwinkle discovered that there were approximately fifty active alkaloid compounds within the plant. With research led by Robert Noble and Charles Thomas Beer, it was found that the rosy periwinkle caused a decrease in the number of white blood cells. They, therefore, speculated that the plant could be effective against cancers in which there was an increased number of white blood cells.

With further work and fractionation, vinblastine was discovered by Noble and Beer at the University of Western Ontario in 1958. Five years later, another alkaloid, known as vincristine, was discovered by J.G. Armstrong and team. Approved by the FDA and later marketed by Eli Lilly and Company, these so-named vinca alkaloids, which had been derived from the rosy periwinkle, proved to be significant discoveries in the battles against Hodgkin's and non-Hodgkin's lymphoma, acute lymphoblastic leukemia (a childhood leukemia), and lung, bladder, and brain cancers.

They are still used today.

As miraculous as this plant has become in the fight against cancer, it is only one of the approximately ten thousand known indigenous plants in Madagascar that has been extensively studied for use in Western medicine. The potential of others remains unknown. With further exploration and study, perhaps there will be many more plants that prove to be beneficial to the human race.

Chapter Five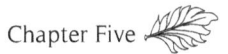

Possibly helpful even with the eradication of cancer, the reversal of dementia, the restoration of sight, the regeneration of neurons and so on.

Mounting an expedition would not be an easy undertaking. The Madagascar trek would consist of several team members who were chosen because of their talents and abilities with film and film production, or science, as well as their ability to get along with others and to work as a team. The members, however, had very little experience with indigenous cultures and remote locations.

The majority of the team would be devoted to the newly established nonprofit, Healing Seekers, and would focus on filming the trek in order to create educational materials. There would also be one scientist working for the for-profit research company, Natural Discoveries, while I would work with both entities.

Both Healing Seekers and Natural Discoveries were newborns. Both were spearheaded by an inexperienced expedition leader and business owner whose only credentials seemed to be a huge heart, unrelenting drive and a deep faith. That was me.

For months I worked with our nonprofit Board to get funding for the trip, and it wasn't long before I realized that fundraising was yet another area in my life where I had no experience. And an area in which I failed miserably. Time after time, my requests for funding were politely rejected or dismissed entirely.

I began to dwell day and night on how the project could be accomplished. Where would we find the funding? How late could I wait to purchase the airline tickets?

How much money did I have in savings?

Friends encouraged me to postpone the trek. But I refused. Maybe it was stubbornness. Maybe it was a crazy belief that everything would somehow work out. Maybe it was a fear of failure.

I wasn't sure.

After months and months of effort, however, we failed to raise one single dollar for the expedition. A fundraiser organized by Board members in an effort to bring in large donors was hugely successful in attendance, but not with securing the needed funding. We were a young organization and unknown, so although it had been a wonderful time, we failed to even cover the evening's expenses.

Frustration and tinges of depression took hold as I realized that one of two things had likely happened. Either we had failed to convince others of the needs of our organization . . . or the very foundation of our organization had been deemed unworthy of support.

The fundraiser had been our last hope. With its failure, I reluctantly agreed to delay the trip one year. But only one year.

With the decision to delay, the pressure immediately lifted. My savings would remain intact and the stress of fundraising was temporarily suspended. Even though there was no longer any immediate anxiety and stress about the trek, I could not sleep that night. My heart was heavy as my feelings shifted from relief and joy to uncertainty and uneasiness. And I could not figure out why.

I thought about the delay in the expedition and even prided myself on the wise decision to do so. Still, something was not right deep within my heart. And then it hit me.

The decision had *not* been the right decision. I had made the decision to delay the trek based on fear—fear of failing to secure the funding, fear of diminishing my savings, fear of not knowing what I was doing. Most of all, I had allowed the decision to override that which was driving my heart.

Chapter Five

I'm not sure how to explain it, but there was no other choice for me than to change my mind. Even though postponing the expedition was a reasonable plan, something stronger was at work. Something deep within was urging me to do it. And to simply trust.

The temporary relief I had experienced earlier from delaying the trip was no match for the peace I felt the moment the expedition was a 'go' once more. It was not going to be comfortable or easy, yet strangely, I felt that if I had said no, a part of me would have died.

The decision to make the trip forced me to step outside of my comfort zone, as it was likely that I would pay for the six-member expedition out of my own pocket. And somehow, that was okay.

My parents raised my brothers and me to work hard to create the lives we wanted. We were taught to buy only those things we could afford and not to go into debt. Growing up, we did not have a lot of the things that many of our friends had, including expensive clothes or cars when we turned sixteen. But what we had had been paid in full.

I had followed this no-debt principle for most of my life, with the exception of my initial car and home. My parents taught us to save for emergencies and retirement and to refrain from using any of the savings unless it was absolutely necessary.

The decision to do the trip would go against all that I had been taught. The decision brought financial instability. And I did not like it.

I continued to question my decision off and on for months. My friends and family also questioned the decision, asking why I wanted to spend all of my vacation time and more importantly, my finances on such a far-fetched notion. Friends gently reminded me that the 'job' I sought did not exist; there were no such positions or salaries for a pharmacist exploring jungles for medicines.

Although their words dampened my spirit and fed my pre-existing doubts and fears, something continued to prod me forward. It was as if a voice deep within my soul was pleading strongly and encouraging me not to let go. Not to give up.

The following months were spent in preparation for Madagascar: researching, planning, lining up interpreters, guides, drivers, airline tickets and lodging, connecting to the Madagascar consulate, getting visas and film permits, while also getting advice from esteemed lemur researchers like Peter Klopfer and Patricia Wright. I also sought guidance and gleaned great insight from Gordon Cragg, former Chief of the Natural Products Branch of the National Cancer Institute, who would later become my friend and mentor.

Whenever possible, I worked extra hours at the pharmacy or as a consultant for my friends at Natural Alternatives in nearby Greensboro to earn additional money. Healing Seekers continued to seek funding and sponsorships for clothing, bags, equipment and for the expedition itself, but to no avail.

Strangely, I felt empowered and in control of my destiny, even though I had great trepidation at what might lie ahead.

When the day came and the team boarded the plane, little did I know, in the days and weeks to come, the depths my heart would feel, the realms my soul would experience and the worlds my eyes would see.

Chapter Six

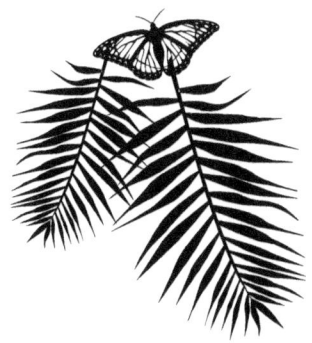

Arriving late at night in Madagascar, we were greeted at the airport by our head guide, Odon. Because of a sudden change in our itinerary made right before we left the United States, our first night in the country would be a short one. By the time we collected our bags and arrived at a small motel, we had only four hours to sleep before we needed to return to the airport to catch an early morning flight.

The spur of the moment decision came two days before our arrival when Odon heard about a village that he thought we would like to visit. Located in a remote northern region, the village was said to be small, simple, isolated and tucked away in the crevice of a bay. The area and its people were completely unknown by Odon and the other guides he knew.

In the Malagasy language, the name of the village sounded like "Nirvana."

And the name alone made me smile.

And the Silent Spoke

Travel to the village began with a flight from the capital city of Antananarivo to Antsiranana, followed by riding several hours in a SUV. Because of our late day arrival to this northern region, we overnighted in a village where visitors and people passing through were often welcomed. The village's small grass huts were quaint and clean, and as we unrolled our sleeping pads and hung mosquito nets above them, the wife of the elder who owned the guest huts announced that she was preparing an evening meal for us.

Outside our huts, a small area had been cleared, and in the middle of it, a large fire blazed much like a bonfire. Near the fire's right outer edge, the owner's wife squatted, stirring the contents of a large dented black pot which sat slightly sideways, nestled in burning wood. As we walked closer to her, she grabbed the pot and held it out for us to see. Inside, liquid broth boiled as parts of a beheaded and plucked chicken peeked through its juices.

She smiled while placing the pot back into the fire's timbers. Then, dipping her left hand into the pot's mixture, she pulled out a large clump of meat and holding it in her hand, cut it into smaller pieces. Tossing the segments back into the pot, she scooted a few feet to her right to attend to a second pot. Lifting its lid, she stirred the white rice before replacing the lid and moving it away from the fire's intense heat.

Although chicken had always been one of my favorites, the sight of gristle, fat, cartilage and other body parts that were tossed back into the pot, and which surfaced each time she stirred, took away much of my appetite. When the plates were distributed and the chicken was passed around, I scooped only the broth from the very top, poured it over a mound of rice and thanked the cook while apologizing for not being very hungry.

Chapter Six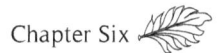

Alec, our sound guy, did the same. The others placed generous portions of both the chicken and rice on their plates. No one, however, enjoyed the gristle.

After dinner, we walked back to our huts. With another early morning start, we decided that before going to sleep, each of us would spend a little time re-organizing our bags and setting out the clothes and equipment that were needed the following day. We would also take turns using the shower stall to rinse off.

Located a hundred feet from our huts and fifty feet from the edge of the forest, the shower was a small, simple wooden structure which provided a nice slow flow of tepid water. Don was the first to bathe, but after he undressed and began to lather, he discovered a snake curled up in one of the corners, only three feet away. With an REI dry towel, which was not large enough to wrap completely around his waist, he ran out of the shower with buttocks exposed, laughing and yelling.

Gathering around him, we laughed while soapy water dripped from his body. With a couple of flashlights, we walked to the shower, poked our heads into the five-foot-by-five-foot structure and tried to determine if the snake was poisonous. A few minutes later, the owner arrived, took a stick, picked up the nonpoisonous snake and carefully returned him to the forest.

The following morning, we left the village for a full day of exploration along the Mozambique Channel. The Channel is located between Madagascar and the eastern coast of Africa. Although our boat driver, Arilova, was in his fifth decade of life, his deep facial wrinkles and prominent white hair made it appear as if he was much older. With strong calloused hands having a texture much like leather, he commanded the boat with confidence and authority.

For hours, we traveled south as the boat surged ahead at full speed, softly skimming the water when it was calm, and when it was rough, going slightly airborne as we catapulted off the waves. It was noisy and difficult to hear one another, so we rode in silence and soaked up the expansiveness. With only a rare siting of a village, the coastline seemed untouched, untainted and astonishingly naturally pure.

To our right seemed an endless sea and to the left, the forest-covered mountainous Madagascar coastline. From the boat, the land mass seemed to be a continuous canopy of green, vibrant and dense vegetation. Its shoreline was narrow and dotted with huge, magnificent boulders.

It was a spectacular day. The sun shone brightly, and the wind blew against my hair . . . slicking it back to the right and then to the left, and back again with each turn of my head. Every so often the boat would hit the water just right and splash its liquid salt over the sides, which cooled and refreshed our bodies. Long after the water had evaporated, I could still taste the salt on my lips.

Pointing to an opening in the shoreline, Arilova yelled of our arrival. Ahead, we could faintly see the signs of a village. I looked back at Odon who gave a nod and grinned.

Nirvana.

From a distance, we could see small moving objects along the beach. At first, there were only a few of them, but with each passing minute the number increased. As we neared, and with the help of our cameras' zoom lenses, it became evident that the objects were people—and the people were children.

The younger ones ran wildly, sprinting toward us near the water's edge only to retreat a few moments later in the direction

Chapter Six

of the village. Their course quickly changed as they zig-zagged up and down the sandy shore. There was no pattern to the frenzy with which they scattered; it was as if their bodies were exploding with surges of energy, impossible to contain. Their excitement was palpable. Even from afar.

As the smaller children darted the coastline, the older ones gathered in groups of three or four, watching our approach. Soon, adults also began to appear.

Nearing the shore, Arilova cut the boat's engine to drift within shouting range. As we waved, Odon walked to the front of the boat and yelled, asking for permission to come ashore. Two elder men walked in our direction. Wading in two feet of water, they smiled and motioned us in.

When the boat reached shallow water, one by one we jumped over the boat's side into two and three feet of water, timing the jumps between the incoming waves. The water was warm and refreshing, blue and crystal clear.

With cameras and equipment held high above our heads, we walked toward the semi-circle of people gathered at the water's edge, directly in front of the boat. Odon and Arilova led the way as we walked toward the two elders who stood in front of the group. After they shook hands with the elders and said hello, we did likewise, greeting them with *"salama,"* meaning 'hello,' and *"misaotra,"* meaning 'thank you.'

Speaking further with the men, Odon asked permission for us to visit the village healer. In order for the request to be granted, Odon and Arilova also had to seek the approval of the other elders, for which they were led away and into the village.

The six of us were told to wait. As we waited, we waved and smiled to the others who had gathered around us. I didn't mind waiting, but it was unfortunate that we could not communicate with them as Odon was our only translator. Eventually, we took out the cameras and the walkie-talkies and played with the children as we attempted to communicate nonverbally.

After almost an hour, far in the distance we saw Odon and Arilova approaching. With them were three men. The spunk in their steps and the smiles on their faces meant only one thing: Nirvana had welcomed us.

Grabbing all of the equipment and gear, we followed the elders to the healer's home. With us was an entourage of children, men and women with whom we continued to laugh as we weaved through the village and around the family huts.

The huts were neat and tidy. Large woven mats were on the ground, and on them, rice, which had been thinly spread to dry in the sun. Women stooped over to sweep away twigs and debris from the areas in front of their huts, using small tied bundles of leaves which they brushed back and forth. Until the ground became a perfectly clean, smooth layer of soil.

As we walked with the villagers, I pointed to a lady's hat and gave a thumbs-up. She took the hat off and gestured for me to put it on. As I did, she snickered while the children burst with laughter. As we walked and played, the only thing heard beyond the giggles coming from their little bodies was the laughter coming from our team.

Many of the children walked with us the twenty minutes it took to reach the outskirts of the village where the healer lived. Arriving at his hut, we learned that he had left early that morning to tend his rice field several miles away but would be returning soon. So, with permission, we waited.

After a couple of hours, we looked down a dirt path to see the figure of a man heading our way. The children announced that he

Chapter Six

was the healer. Of short stature, he was thin and appeared to be close to thirty years of age. His youth was surprising because other healers I had met in my life had been more advanced in age. It was intriguing that in such youth he had earned the respect of his community as their healer.

Greeting him, Odon introduced the team and then asked permission for us to have an audience with him.

The healer's name was Jahiry. He gave little eye contact, and his words were soft spoken and few. Surprisingly, his demeanor was rather cool and distant, completely opposite that of other healers I had met. My team members appeared to be just as bewildered by the unresponsiveness and lack of warmth, yet like me, stood quiet and still, as Odon continued to carry most of the conversation.

My mind raced. Maybe we were not as welcomed as I had thought. Maybe he objected to our unexpected visit. Maybe he had never had interactions with outsiders. Or maybe, just maybe, he was shy and introverted.

Regardless, not once did I detect any level of geniality, which conflicted with everything that we had experienced since our arrival to the village. And to the country. No matter how hard I tried to grasp his nonverbal cues, I could not. It was not fear that I felt, but uneasiness at not knowing what to think or feel.

After a few minutes, Jahiry looked at me, smiled ever so slightly, nodded and then motioned for us to follow. He led us down a dirt path to an isolated wooden hut. Only a few feet surrounding the structure had been cleared, leaving the area beyond it overgrown with tall grass. Five feet behind the hut was a wooden fence which separated the building from the forest.

The hut was like others we had seen in the village, resting upon stilts that raised it a foot off the ground. Two wooden steps led to a small, narrow and unpainted front door. The rest of the tiny building was painted green, except for one single strip of white paint which ran horizontally along the bottom two feet at its base.

There were no other people or structures within sight.

Jahiry stepped up to the door, stopped momentarily, and then motioned for us to follow. Before entering, Odon slipped off his sandals, and we did the same.

Inside, the room was dark except for tiny slivers of light which entered through the cracks in the walls and a small amount of light which came through the door. There were no windows or any other openings. The room was so small that it was impossible for all of us, the cameras and equipment to fit, so three members of our six-member team had to remain outside where they stuck their heads just inside the doorway.

For the Malagasy people, the four directions within a dwelling or structure have significant meaning. The East represents the sacred, the ancestors and the dead. The West represents the common or ordinary life; and it is typically the West where a door is placed. An additional door might also be placed on the East side, but that door would only be used to carry out the deceased.

The North represents honor and it is the area in which the head of the household sits and sleeps. The South represents the impure. It would be the area that animals occupy.

Jahiry sat on an old wooden stool, which raised him only a few inches off the floor. Sitting with his back to us, he faced east. We were told to sit behind him.

Wrapped in a white cloth from his waist to his knees, Jahiry's exposed upper body made visible several deep scars across his back. The only eye contact he gave was when he turned his head slightly in response to Odon.

Chapter Six

In front of Jahiry was a small wooden table that served as an altar. Objects covered the table and hung on the wall behind it—bowls, knives, plants, rocks—and three small mirrors that were aged with etched black markings and had limited visibility. The mirrors were propped up side by side on the table, leaning against the wall in front of him and reflecting that which was behind him.

The bowls, plants and rocks were things I had read about and even seen in South America, items that were used by many healers around the world as sacred objects. But the knives caught me off guard. They looked much like Bowie knives and hung on the wall in front of him. Within his reach.

On the floor to his left was a small bundle of plants, leaves and stems. Known as the *"zoro firarazana,"* or the 'corner of prayers,' this northeast corner of the hut, according to Odon, was regarded as the most sacred space, for it was considered hallowed for the ancestors.

The walls of the hut were constructed of a bamboo-like material. Large red cloths partially covered three of them. Red, Jahiry explained, because that is the favorite color of God.

The cloth that hung directly in front of him had symbols painted in white—a star, a dot with a circle around it, and a crescent shaped moon. They were images of celestial bodies, Odon translated, which represented the 'highest places' for it was only in the highest places where God and the spirits dwelled.

I asked many questions and he softly answered. There was little elaboration. Not only did it take time to translate the Malagasy into English, it also took time to understand the meaning behind his words.

Jahiry treated people with medicinal plants, yet he first tried to heal them spiritually with the help of ancestral spirits. As a young boy, Jahiry had been visited by spirits, who told him that the people of his village needed him to be their healer and that he had already been chosen by a particular spirit who would help and guide him. Accepting the role as a healer, Jahiry became a medium through which the spirits could speak, guiding and directing him in helping others.

As a spiritual healer, he helped members of his community with emotional issues, bad fortunes, curses and with advice and guidance on marriage, crops and other issues. As a physical healer, he diagnosed problems and prescribed local medicinal plants and remedies.

Known as an *ombiasa*, Jahiry communicated with the spirit world, summoning ancestors for their guidance to help him heal the people in his village. He excelled over the years as an ombiasa, working not only with the initial spirit who had chosen him, but with fourteen other spirits. During a session, however, only one spirit would be present at a time.

Many of the ancestral spirits were of royalty and nobility, while others were deceased military or common people. Depending on the problem that a person was facing, Jahiry would call upon the spirit that was best suited to help. The practice of calling on a particular spirit reminded me of the Catholic church's practice of seeking help from a specific patron saint.

For Jahiry, it was as if the spirits were at his beck and call.

Although Jahiry was an ombiasa, there were other healers known as troombas. Instead of a having a conversation with a spirit like Jahiry did, a troomba was a man or woman who actually embodied the spirit. In other words, a troomba allowed the spirit to take possession of his or her body.

Chapter Six

In the moment a spirit embodied the man or woman, his or her body would begin shaking, swaying or experiencing some sort of rapid or jerky body movements. After a few minutes, the movements would cease, and a completely different personality would emerge. This new persona would often be in stark contrast to the normal voice, tone and disposition of the man or woman.

To accommodate the embodied spirit, the troomba would first change into special clothes that were to be worn only when the spirit was present. Often this was a man's white shirt or other masculine clothing. And sometimes there would be an accessory like a hat.

The spirit typically would have a beverage like alcohol or a drink which looked to be a cloudy mixture of white clay and water. Beverages were said to be pleasing to the spirits and the beverage that the troomba sipped throughout the session was said to be the spirit's beverage of choice.

At the end of a session, the man or woman embodying the spirit would once again shake, sway, move or shiver, until the spirit departed the body. The healer would then slowly remove the special clothing and, in a daze, sit quietly before needing to rest.

I had read about these practices before going to Madagascar and in theory, I got them. Or so I thought. As an ombiasa, Jahiry was able to communicate with the spirit world to guide him to treat the physical, mental and emotional problems of others. A stomach issue, for example, was treated with honey, clay and coconuts. The coconuts had to be pulled directly off the tree and not taken from the ground.

If a person was possessed or bothered by bad spirits, the knives were used. As an ombiasa, Jahiry would invoke one of the ancestral spirits who would then, through him, use the knives to rid and kill any evil spirit. Although I questioned what the practice entailed, Jahiry gave little detail other than to say the knives would eliminate the problem.

As I was trying to wrap my head around all of it, Odon asked if he might ask Jahiry's help with a problem he was having at home. Agreeing to do so would require the healer to go into ceremony to seek the advice and guidance of one of the spirits.

It was a great opportunity to not only help Odon, but to also witness firsthand this healing practice. Known as a *fivoriana,* the ceremony was sacred, and as such, filming was prohibited. Furthermore, only two of us were allowed to stay with Odon and Jahiry.

Thinking that we would perhaps be allowed to still record the audio, Alec, our sound guy, was chosen to join me. Even though we soon learned that sound recordings were also forbidden during a ceremony, Alec remained.

While the other members of the team stepped away from the hut, Jahiry closed the door halfway and instructed us to turn around and face the door, which was west. No one was permitted to face east, the sacred direction. Not even him. We were told to sit, with legs crossed, knee-to-knee across the width of the room. The hut was so small that in this position our knees had to slightly overlap in order for the four of us to fit.

Each of us was then given a narrow strip of thick red cloth, and we were told to put it on as a blindfold. Doing so made it impossible to detect anyone or anything or even a glimmer of light. Jahiry then completely closed the wooden door.

To my right sat Odon and to his right (within my arm's reach) was Jahiry. Alec was to my left. Two feet in front of us was the door, which separated us from the other members of our team.

The four of us sat quietly. Not a word was spoken.

After a few minutes of silence, Jahiry spoke loudly and briefly

Chapter Six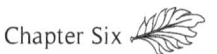

in Malagasy. And burped. Then, more silence. Odon whispered that the healer was calling the spirit.

After another five minutes, Jahiry again spoke what seemed to be the same words. And then more silence.

We sat. We waited. No sound could be heard, not even the wind outside.

Suddenly, without warning, the entire hut began to shake, and the door and table rattled. It felt like an earthquake tremor, which slightly jarred our bodies. And then, from behind us, a voice materialized as if from thin air. It was loud and harsh, deep and boisterous. It was eerie and unlike any voice I had ever heard. Not human—and yet, I could not imagine the form from which it came. It reminded me of voices of demonic entities depicted in horror movies, combined with the gruff, raspy sounds made from an old Victrola record player whose record is finished.

The voice, moreover, seemed to be coming from over my left shoulder. It was as if the entity was directly behind Alec and me.

I was afraid to move. I was almost afraid to breathe. I had never in my life heard such a voice or feared such a darkness. I pressed my knee into Alec's, and he pressed back. At the same time, I silently asked God and the angels for protection over both of us.

Jahiry began to talk and Odon whispered the translations. Odon quietly explained the problem he was having with his rice field. For several weeks someone had been stealing his rice and because food was scarce, the rice that had been stolen was making it difficult for Odon to feed his family.

More than five hundred kilos were missing. With no idea who was stealing it, Odon decided to seek the aid of the ombiasa and the spirit.

Jahiry spoke to the spirit for what seemed to be several minutes in a language other than Malagasy, and when he stopped, the spirit began. After each response from the spirit, Jahiry would talk to Odon, and Odon would then lean toward Alec and me and softly translate.

Jahiry asked Odon, "How long has this been going on? How much rice? Do you have any enemies?" With the answers, he would return to the conversation with the spirit.

The conversations went on for at least half an hour. The spirit eventually asked that Odon return at a later time and bring an offering. At that point he would be told what to do.

Odon then turned to Alec and me and asked if we had any questions for the spirit. The only thing we could muster was a quiet "No thank you." It was the first time I had ever been with a traditional healer and didn't have a lot of questions. And it was the first time I ever looked forward to the closing of a ceremony or the end of a conversation.

Jahiry spoke once more to the spirit and after that, there was a short period of silence. And then, as in the beginning, the entire hut shook, and the door and table rattled.

And the spirit was gone.

We lifted the blindfolds, and Jahiry got up and opened the door. Standing a few feet on the other side, staring at us was the rest of the team. As we emerged from the hut, they gathered closer to us while Jahiry walked back to his home, which was a good seventy-five yards away.

They had been stunned to see the door of the hut shaking both times, not knowing what we were doing inside. They had heard Jahiry's and Odon's voices, yet surprisingly never heard the loud, boisterous voice of the spirit. This, I simply could not understand. The walls of the hut were thin and the spaces between the bamboo material allowed small rays of light and air to enter. The spirit's

Chapter Six

voice should have easily penetrated as well as the other voices, especially being so thundering and intense.

Yet, it did not.

My teammates Olivia, Gary and Eduardo had been sitting outside the hut, fifteen yards away, while Don sat behind the hut, leaning against the fence and catching up on his notes. No one had seen a soul, not even an animal.

Still shaking inside, my voice quivered as I spoke. My breath was short and sporadic, having to stop several times to gather myself. Alec's face was bright rosy red and his breathing shallow, as he too tried to explain and make sense of it all.

Gary and Eduardo discretely walked closer to the hut. Getting on their hands and knees, they peered underneath the structure before walking around its perimeter, looking closely for some explanation of the shaking and the presence of another entity.

After several minutes they whispered to each other and then looked back at the rest of us and shrugged. They could not see a way for anyone or anything to have entered the hut without going through the front door. There were no windows and, apart from the door, there were no openings. The roof could only be accessed by some sort of ladder, and the walls and floor were solidly built.

Odon later explained that connections to the spirit world were very deep and real, and the practice of seeking help from the spirits was very common in Madagascar. For them, it was as normal as it was for us in the United States to seek aid from a doctor or guidance from a minister or priest, clairvoyant or psychic.

As we listened, we began to better grasp the beauty and the sacredness of the ombiasa practice. While we walked back to Jahiry's home, the discussions about the spirit world continued. Aloud, I questioned my own spiritual practices and my failure to discover the extents and depths of my connections to God and the angels, who I believed were ceaseless in watching over me. Others expressed similar thoughts.

The ancestral spirit which had appeared that day had at one time been a high-ranking military official in his earthly life, which helped explain the intensity and abrasiveness of his voice. Nevertheless, it took a while for our heart rates to slow and the flushing in Alec's face to subside.

The spirit's surreal, inhuman voice, however, would stay with me for months.

The global practices of worshiping and honoring one's God and spiritual beings are as varied as the cultures themselves. For some, being baptized in a pool of water might be unusual. For others, speaking in tongues. And yet for others, an ombiasa who calls upon ancestral spirits or a troomba who embodies them.

I will never forget that day in the village that our team continued to call Nirvana. It not only gave me greater insight into the lives of those who welcomed us . . . but it also welcomed me into a new and expanded realm of my own Nirvana.

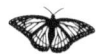

Chapter Seven

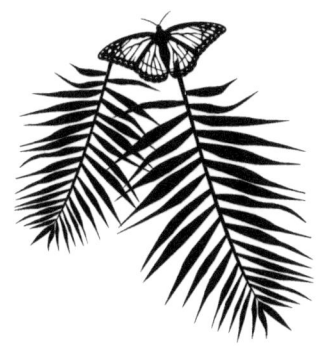

She paused, took a deep breath and slowly exhaled. In the moment of silence, a cell phone rang. It was something that had happened several times during the day. Each time one rang, the niece or nephew would politely excuse herself or himself, leave the room and answer it. She didn't mind as she knew their lives were busy, filled with family, work and other obligations.

Although she was enjoying the time with them immensely, she was tired. The day had brought a lot of activity, and she had talked more than she had in months.

Noticing her silence and obvious fatigue, the cousins jumped right in with conversations about a multitude of things. They reminisced about their childhood, the mischief and the trouble they had gotten into and the fun and the games they had played. They spoke of their marriages and raising children, their social lives and careers . . . and both the pleasures and difficulties thereof. And of the dreams they still held.

For her, it was lovely to simply listen. As they spoke, she recalled moments when they were young, running free and laughing hysterically. She let her mind wander as a spectacular slideshow began to flash *throughout her mind, movie clips of memories and special moments with them that had spanned decades. And yet, it felt more like months.*

She remembered when they all fit within the cockpit of one of her father's white-water kayaks, screaming with excitement as the boat slid across the lawn, pulled by one of her brothers. And when they would crawl onto her father's back as he knelt on all fours and pretended to be a bucking bronco, or when they would run and jump into her mother's arms. She also remembered their tiny arms around her neck and their fingers wrapped around one of hers. She remembered their soft skin and the scent of baby powder.

She could still see the children within, even though the bodies and voices that now surrounded her were dramatically different from those of years past. She could not be prouder. Or love them more.

The smell of homemade lasagna, one of their favorites, radiated throughout the room and was followed shortly by the aroma of fresh baked bread. Dinner also included organic salad with goat cheese, topped off by her mother's special balsamic dressing, made of olive oil, sugar, balsamic and celery salt.

To complement the meal, and for their enjoyment throughout the weekend, a variety of beverages was made available. A selection of wines, Red Oak beer and a full bar at their disposal. In the weeks prior to their arrival, she had meticulously marked the finest bottles of wine in the cellar for them to savor.

Collected over forty-five years, the bottles had been reserved for life's special moments. Yet, they had remained untouched, for the joy of such celebrations had ceased the day her partner died.

The weekend, however, would present the perfect occasion for serving only the most cherished.

Chapter Seven

Although she longed to stay awake, exhaustion hit its peak. Sinking a little further into her soft leather chair, she closed her eyes, tilted her head slightly, and rested.

And could not be happier.

Hours later, she awakened to her niece covering her with a warm, soft blanket, tucking its edges tightly around her.

Thank you.

I think I'll just sleep here tonight. You know, it wasn't that long ago that I was tucking you into bed. How I wish I had done that more often.

I love you.

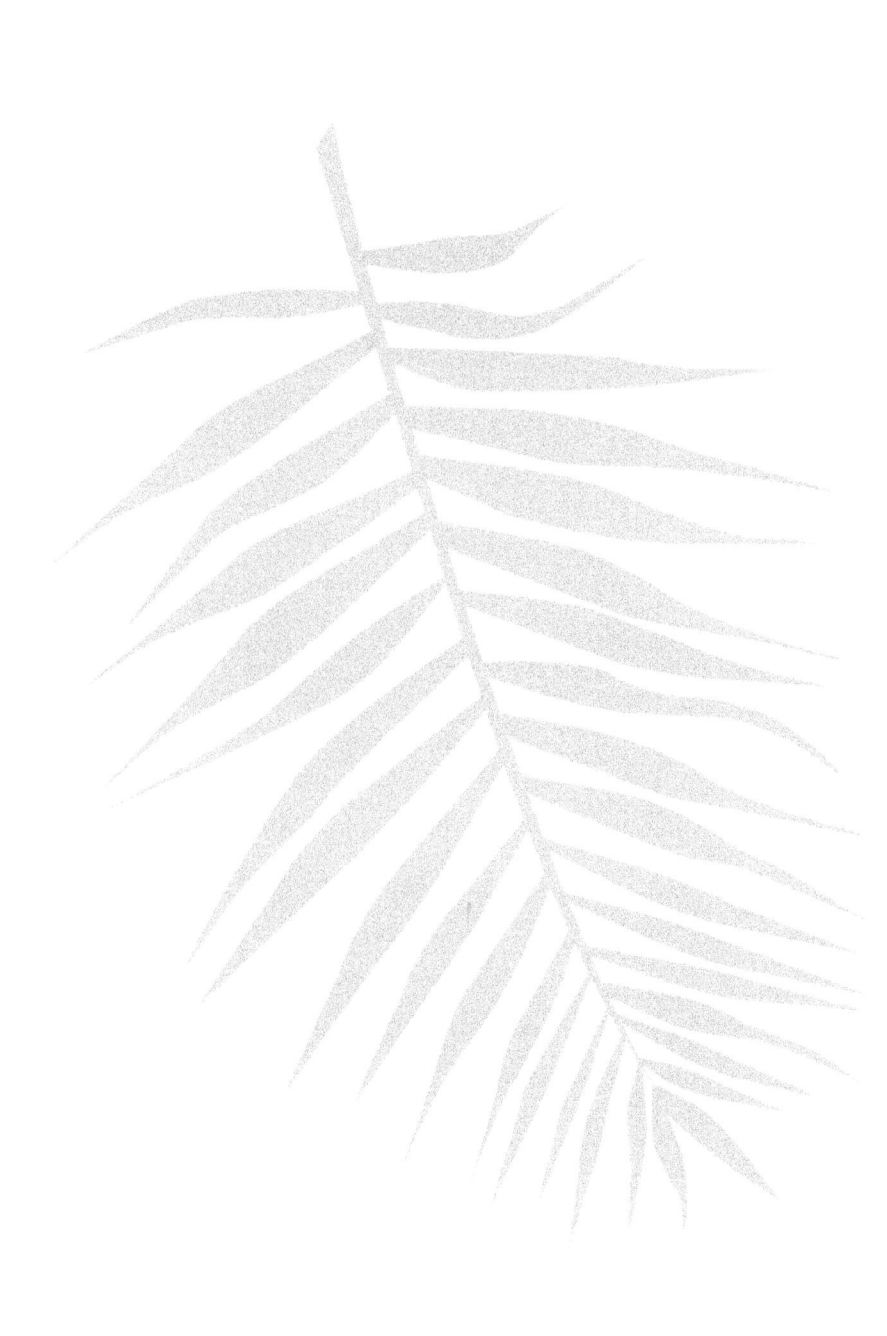

Chapter Eight

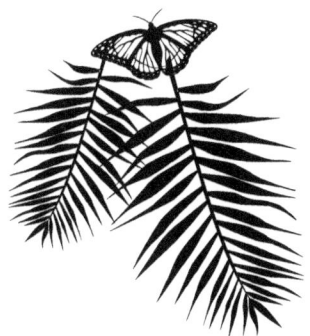

The smell of coffee had always been a wonderful way to start her day. Although it had been another restless night with little sleep, she was happy and eager to spend every possible moment with her nieces and nephews . . . her kids.

One by one, they had awakened and joined her, cradling cups of hot tea and coffee. The room smelled of hazelnut and vanilla from their lattes, and of cinnamon from the freshly baked Moravian sugar cake made from the recipe shared by her dear friend Jesse.

She knew her time with them was limited and the weekend would quickly pass, so she wasted no time with small talk.

You were extremely blessed to have the grandparents you had. The closeness. And unconditional love.

Grandparents are cherished all over the world, yet in our Western society we have greatly diminished their value. Honor and respect have often been replaced with dismissal and irreverence as the family unit continues its demise. The failure to utilize elders' wisdom and experience has resulted in hindered growth and progress in numerous areas . . . including business. Problems and failures that have emerged would likely have been avoided had such guidance been sought. And heeded.

In other cultures, however, the elderly are heralded as advisers and the keepers of great wisdom. They are coveted for their insight and guidance as well as for their love and protection.

Almost two years after the Madagascar trip, we traveled to Papua New Guinea. Like Madagascar, it is known for its tremendous bio-diversity. And with hundreds of indigenous groups, Papua New Guinea is known as the most heterogeneous country in the world.

The expedition's itinerary would involve travel to four different regions, mandating considerable time because of the limited roads, airstrips and other means of transportation. It would take, for example, a flight and then almost a full day in an SUV just to reach the KukuKuku tribe located in the higher elevations of the Morobe province. To spend four days to travel to and from a destination was a big decision, and twice I almost canceled that leg of the trip. Time was precious and every day spent in an SUV, boat or airplane was a day that seemed unproductive.

But few outsiders traveled there. And that made all the difference.

It was an arduous journey from Lae to the home of the KukuKuku tribe, located in the southwest area of the province. And it required

Chapter Eight

great patience. Although the roads were partially paved, they were rough and bumpy with potholes, often as wide as the road. Unlike our driver, Raims, an inexperienced driver would mean vehicle damage and flat tires. Although we were in the dry season, we were told by Raims that during the rainy season, sections were so muddy that they became impassable.

I'd heard little about Menyamya and the KukuKuku (or Angu) people, other than they smoked the bodies of their dead and that the region still had unconfirmed reports of cannibalism. The cannibalism intrigued me not because of an infatuation with the practice, but because it represented a rawness of life and a practice untouched by the outside world. To glimpse such a life that was so different from my own, even from a distance, was exciting.

Pointing to an unmarked area on the map, Raims estimated that it would take between ten and twelve hours by SUV to reach the isolated village. The trip was risky, as we had no idea if we would be allowed to enter the land after traveling so far. There were no phones, radios or internet to ask permission ahead of time, and my mind raced with the stories I had heard of outsiders being rejected from tribal lands (sometimes harshly).

I couldn't help but to think of Michael Rockefeller, the son of Nelson Rockefeller. In 1961, Michael had traveled to the southern Netherlands New Guinea on an expedition to collect art for Harvard's Peabody Museum of Archaeology and Ethnology. When his small boat capsized, Michael swam toward the shore but was never seen again.

Some people believe that Michael never made it to shore, but instead drowned or was killed by sharks or some other predator. Most, however, believe that he was killed by an indigenous tribe, who sacrificed him in order to help atone for the deaths of their tribal members who had been killed earlier by another 'tribe,' the Dutch patrol. The Dutch patrol, like Michael, were members of the 'white tribe.'

Michael weighed heavily in my thoughts; yet even though my mind told me to exercise caution and to be alert, my heart believed that at its core, mankind was good and that we would be fine.

Travel was at a slow pace. Frequently, Raims hit the brakes suddenly, swerving to dodge yet another deep hole in the road before accelerating again. He seemed to hit the brakes just in time to avoid a hard hit, causing our bodies to slam into one another and into the bags and gear that surrounded us, making us laugh as if we were children on a carnival ride.

On either side of the road was flourishing jungle with foliage so thick it would take enormous energy to cut through even a short distance. I looked at my five team members, three of whom—Eduardo, Don and Alec—were members of the team in Madagascar while the other two, environmentalists, ocean conservationists and friends, Simone and Felix, were on their first trip with us. As the expedition leader, I realized that I was responsible for each of them. They were not only team members; they were my friends. What if something happened to one of them? Or to all of us? Who would search for us or even know where to begin?

Our guide Sabby chatted nonstop about the famous mummies of Menyamya. A man of short stature and in his early thirties, he was energetic yet insecure as he hesitated to make decisions or even give an opinion. The mummies, however, excited him, and in broken English he spoke of the bodies, which were smoked and then carried

Chapter Eight

to their permanent resting place on a cliff. He warned us to be careful as the cliff was steep, and a fall could be fatal. He explained that the area was sacred, revered by the KukuKuku people so much that he hoped the elders would allow us, as outsiders, to enter.

After a while, we realized that Sabby's excessive giddiness was due to the stories he had been told, not from personal experience, as it was the first time he or any of our guides had seen the mummies. In fact, it was the first time any of them had traveled to this region of the country.

Although we were still many hours from the Menyamya village, it was getting dark and we needed to stop for the evening. Thankfully Sabby had been given the name of a landowner whom he believed would allow us to stay on his land overnight. Pitching camp on another's property without permission was not only disrespectful, but ill-considered.

As the last bit of daylight was fading, we arrived at the small community where the landowner was said to live. Alongside the road were fifteen to twenty small huts. In front of the huts, men and women sat around fires while children played further away. The village was one of only a few that we had seen on that day.

Raims slowed to ask a lone man walking beside the road the location of the landowner's hut. Following the directions, Raims drove another fifty yards before veering off onto a dirt path. The path was barely wide enough for a vehicle and was surrounded on either side with dense overgrowth. Two hundred yards further, he stopped in front of a single hut, cut off the engine and, with Sabby, went in search of the landowner. A few minutes later they returned with the elder.

With bare feet, loose brown pants and an oversized beige shirt, the owner radiated kindness and gentleness. His brown eyes sparkled as his deep facial lines and wrinkles seemed to expand with his smile. While shaking each of our hands, he extended an invitation to stay in his guesthouse.

The guesthouse was a gracious offer. The rooms, simple and clean, were bare except for an inch-thick mattress that looked more like a sleeping pad. Directly over the center of each mattress and hanging from the ceiling was a bundled mosquito net. Untying the cord that held it together would allow the bulk of the net to drop below.

Taking my bags to one of the rooms, I closed the wooden door, released the net, and then tucked three of its edges underneath the corners of the sleeping pad. Before tucking in the fourth corner, I crawled inside the net. Throwing my bivy sack on top of the mattress, I rolled up my Gore-Tex jacket, placed it at the head of the bed as a pillow and stretched out.

The trip to Menyamya was taking much longer than originally anticipated. Because Sabby had no prior experience with the region, his calculations turned out to be considerably inaccurate. The following day would bring yet another full day of bumpy travel as we were only a little over half way there, and still many hours away. I couldn't help but wonder if traveling to this area had been the right decision. It was consuming much more time than I had imagined, and I prayed it would be worth it.

Early the next morning, I was the first one up and made a direct path to a large room where the landowner had arranged to have hot water for our coffee. It was only on treks that I found instant coffee decadent.

After the first cup, I savored the mango, pineapple and crackers that his wife had graciously provided for breakfast. The flavors of

Chapter Eight

the fruit were extraordinary, and I had become quite addicted to the crackers. Two-inch-by-two-inch, the square crackers were thick with a crunchy outer layer and came in a variety of flavors. The cheese and beef flavors were good, but it was the chicken flavor that I found impossible to resist.

Gradually, the others joined me. Last to arrive was Sabby. Grabbing a chunk of pineapple, he straddled the wooden bench to my left and said, "There's been early rain. The road may be bad. We may not be able to drive it. There's no way to get a report—we have to find out ourselves."

My heart sank. After spending all of this time traveling, the thought of not reaching the village was crushing. I felt a tinge of frustration and irritation forming deep within, but I suppressed it.

We finished breakfast and thanked our host once more, giving him a generous monetary gift. Within the hour, all of our bags were loaded into the SUV, and we were on our way. It wasn't long before the dry dirt became moist and the moistened soil became mud. Regardless of Raims' skill, the vehicle often slid uncontrollably as if it was on a sheet of ice.

Ironically, we found the ride fun and yelled with excitement like a bunch of kids on an amusement park ride, knowing that Raims would soon have it under control. Enjoying the accolades, Raims laughed as he accelerated and braked a little harder than necessary to make it more entertaining.

But then the level landscape in which we were traveling changed. And with it, the enjoyment stopped. The rolling hills gave way to mountains with spectacular overlooks and drops. The flat road became a steep, winding, narrow path that looked more like the trail of a serpent, slithering its way through the rugged terrain.

And the Silent Spoke

Wide enough for only one vehicle, the road hugged the mountainside. With no guard rails or protection, sliding off the road and down the mountain was foremost in my thoughts.

The anxiety was palpable, and we all leaned forward with eyes focused ahead. No one spoke.

There is something about not having control over a situation that compounds fear. There was nothing to do but to pray and to trust the experience and decisions of our driver. It didn't help, however, that Raims had never been on the road before and had no idea which areas were known to wash out during heavy rains . . . areas, which he had heard, could sweep away the heaviest of vehicles.

As we traveled, Raims occasionally stopped the vehicle so that he, Sabby and another guide could more closely inspect the road. Their sandals sank into the mud, causing them to slip and slide. Walking the road ahead, they scouted beyond blind bends, determining which side was the safer side of the road to hug. In areas that were extremely slick, they spread grass and sticks on top of the mud to help with traction.

We had two choices: one was to keep moving forward; the second was to go back. But to go back would require driving in reverse for a good distance as there was no place to turn the vehicle around. Raims was willing to do either, so the decision ultimately rested on me as the leader. Despite how frightening the road that lay ahead seemed, it was the thought of going back in reverse on the slick mud that made my stomach turn upside down.

My mind raced. First, there was the safety of the team and our guides. Second, there was the issue of damaging the vehicle, which could leave us stranded for weeks waiting on repair parts or another vehicle. Third, if we got through to the village and the rains continued, we could be stranded in the village for up to a month, which would be devastating to the rest of the expedition.

Chapter Eight

Everyone remained silent. No one complained. Finally, I asked if anyone felt that we should turn around and close this chapter of the trek. But as I suspected, regardless of the angst and unease with moving forward, the unanimous response was to keep moving forward unless the driver or guides insisted otherwise.

I gripped the underside of my seat. With every turn and with every slide, I grasped so tightly that my knuckles turned white. Twice, the vehicle slid within inches of a drop off, but we continued on . . . creeping at a nominal speed as the road twisted and turned, going up and down in elevation.

Finally, the terrain began to level out. And with it, the treacherous mountain pass slowly faded behind us.

Relieved, I let go of the seat and grabbed our most favorite dry bag, which had been filled with bite size Snickers, Baby Ruths, Kit Kats and Butterfingers. Passing the heavy orange bag around, everyone grabbed a treat, and shortly thereafter the laughter returned. Even Raims, who had never had the candy from the United States, released his grip on the wheel long enough to grab a Snickers. And then a Baby Ruth.

It was another hour before we saw huts lining the sides of the road. From first glance, the village seemed to be small with the ten to fifteen huts near the road; however, Sabby told us that many members of a community live away from such a road, and it is, therefore, always difficult to predict its actual size. As we slowed to pass through, people stopped what they were doing, turned and looked. We waved, but they didn't wave back. They stood motionless. Even the children.

And stared.

Something didn't feel right. Perhaps it was the way the villagers were looking at us. The smiles and waves that had been returned when we had passed through other villages, were absent. Instead, our greetings were met with bewildered stares and puzzled looks.

Suddenly from out of the silence and from behind our vehicle were loud yells, almost as if someone was saying, "Hey you!" We turned and looked out the back window to see several men running after us. I looked at Raims in front of me and could see his facial expressions in the rearview mirror. His brow was furrowed, and his eyes were moving from the rearview mirror—to the road ahead—to Sabby, who was sitting in the passenger seat beside him. He seemed unsettled and hesitant, first braking slightly at the sound of the yells and then slowly accelerating. I didn't know if Raims and Sabby understood the words or if it was the harsh tones of the yelling that rattled them.

Accelerating slightly, Raims only further provoked the men, who responded with even louder yells and more annoyed inflections. Glancing over at Sabby (who remained speechless), he pressed on the brake and stopped. His full attention then turned to the outside rearview mirror. Leaning forward, he stared at the reflection of the men running up from behind the vehicle. Running closely behind them were other men, women and children.

Within moments our SUV was encircled by a crowd standing three, four and five deep. Pushing each other in attempts to get closer, several young men thrust their heads into our windows to look around inside, coming within inches of our own faces. Smiling, we inconspicuously covered up equipment and bags and used our bodies to limit their view of our belongings. This was

Chapter Eight

not something we had done before, but the moment they began to gather around the SUV, Sabby ordered us to do it.

Later he would explain that there were stories of bags and belongings being grabbed and a person then being forced to buy them back at great expense—or worse, the robbers running off with the goods . . . never to be seen again. Clothing and food were one thing, but the cameras and equipment, visas, money, and medical kits were another.

We nervously smiled at the ever-increasing crowd as we waved our hands and said, *"Moning nau,"* which meant 'hello/good morning' in the Tok Pisin language, only to be met with confused looks and a language we did not understand. Meanwhile, the men who had yelled at us to stop, gathered outside the two front doors. Pressing their bodies against the doors, they stuck their heads slightly inside the vehicle's open windows.

The men were older than the others in the crowd, and the authority with which they spoke implied that they were men of power within the village. Their expressions and the tones of their voices were jarring. Even without translations, it was obvious they were upset.

Raims and Sabby physically pulled away from the heads which protruded inside their windows, until they were both leaning on the vehicle's center console. With either blank stares or with expressions of fear or shock, they glanced frequently at one another, but said very little. When they did speak to the men, they did so weakly.

Our predicament was too intense for any of us to ask for translations and explanations. The gestures and tones in their voices, however, spoke volumes.

We were not in a good situation.

Raims released his foot from the brake and slowly moved forward, hoping to disengage; however, the instant he did, one of the men (perhaps the village chief, as he seemed to be the leader) yelled louder than ever, causing Raims to immediately stop the vehicle.

My mind raced. Even though we had never been in this area, other outsiders had. And it was possible that the village's previous experience with outsiders was now influencing their interactions with us. Perhaps too, the village had simply heard unfavorable stories about people like us.

Sabby eventually turned to us and said that the men wanted to know what we were doing, where we were going and why. They either didn't want us here or they were looking for some kind of payment which would allow us to pass through. It could also be a demonstration of the power they had within the village and of their authority, he said, in which the men would later be exalted by the other members of the tribe for standing up to the "white clan."

After several minutes, Sabby offered a monetary gift, which was eagerly accepted. We were then allowed to pass through.

I didn't believe the village intended to harm us, but rather, they wanted to protect the land and village through which we were trespassing. It was the first time, however, that I had to pay an indigenous tribe for passage. Thoughts flooded my mind. Money had more power in these remote areas of the world than I had ever imagined.

In hindsight, the incident with the village was no different than other situations in the world, where tolls are collected on turnpikes, identifications are required to enter corporate lands and businesses . . . and private communities, fees are paid for park entrances, and passports are necessary for entries into foreign territories.

Chapter Eight

For an hour and a half afterward, we continued traveling along the road as it progressively became more difficult to traverse. It was in ill repair and without four-wheel drive would have been impossible to navigate. At one point, we had to cross a forty-foot bridge made up of wooden planks, some of which were broken and rotten. Off the right side of the bridge was a fifty-foot drop into the jungle and off the other side, a ten-foot drop into a rock filled stream.

After several minutes debating the situation, Raims and Sabby decided to move forward even with the weight of occupants, bags and equipment. We suggested getting out and walking across, but Sabby insisted that we were fine.

Slowly, Raims navigated the boards and hugged the left side, staying as far away as possible from the steep right embankment. The creaky boards moaned and slightly gave way. But did not break.

Safely on the other side, he drove another fifteen minutes before pulling off to the side of the road. Ahead of us, the road transformed into coarse, jagged terrain that was more like an incomplete, abandoned path than a road. Winding up the left side of the path was a crevice, twelve inches deep and fifteen inches wide, which looked as if it had been formed by a small river running through it. The left and right sides of the path were uneven, varying two to three feet in elevation, which made Raims too nervous to have any passengers, for fear that the SUV would topple over. Continuing alone, he drove ahead as we proceeded on foot.

As we began to walk, several children came out of the surrounding woods. Their appearance surprised us. We had not seen any recent signs of village life and were startled that anyone knew that we were there. Saying hello in Tok Pisin, we smiled and waved as they came nearer. We communicated with simple sentences in English while the children spoke a language unknown to our guides. Using hand gestures and the words Menyamya, Angu and KukuKuku, we learned that the path ahead led to the Angu chief.

Within minutes of hiking, we were surrounded by more than twenty children as well as several adults, who seemed excited and eager for the adventure. A small group of young boys perhaps six to eight years of age gathered around me. The further we walked and the more we smiled at one another, the closer they came, until they were within a few inches. Putting my arms around the shoulders of the two closest to me caused them to burst into laughter.

Those two remained by my side for the duration of the walk.

At one point, a young teenage girl ran in front of me, turned around, and walking backwards, tried to communicate. Even though I could not understand her language and she could not understand mine, she noticed that I kept glancing at the top of her head, where a baby chicken was resting. The chick was perfectly balanced and comfortably cushioned in her hair as if riding in a plush carriage. Reaching up, she fed the chick a small insect—and seeing my delight, did it once again.

All around us, the children ran, snickered and laughed. Their bodies moved with smooth and fluid agility, their bare feet seemingly impervious to the rocks and hard terrain. The clothing they wore were mixtures of beautiful fabrics, styles and colors. There were no apparent consistencies in the clothing like in Western society, where the majority of children, for example, might wear blue jeans. It was as if it didn't matter what colors or patterns were mixed as long as they served the purpose of covering the body.

Although the path had a steady incline and we walked a good distance, we were so enthralled with the children that we paid little attention to the time or effort. When we reached the top of the hill, however, we abruptly stopped.

Chapter Eight

In front of us, a man-made barrier composed of plant material stretched across the path. The only other structures that I had seen within indigenous communities in other parts of the world were fences built to contain livestock. Such a barricade blatantly signaled 'private' and 'do not enter.'

Upon closer inspection, the structure appeared to serve more like a curtain. But instead of cloth, its drapes were made of long stringy vines, covered in leaves and debris that allowed a small amount of transparency through to the other side.

The curtain of organic matter dangled from pieces of timber, crafted from small tree limbs tied end to end, that functioned as a curtain rod. Suspended ten feet above the ground, the wooden beam extended fifty to sixty feet across.

As we neared the barrier, the children and other villagers quietly backed off and stepped to the side, allowing us to proceed alone. I walked in front of the others and felt unsettled, even though Sabby motioned for me to continue.

I worried we were trespassing on sacred or forbidden land. If the people of the village were not continuing and perhaps were not permitted, why should we be?

With the other team members only feet behind, I walked toward the middle of the structure where it was less dense and appeared to be an entrance. Then, I briefly turned around to look at Sabby and Raims once more for guidance. But they too had remained behind, standing near the children and other villagers. Although they seemed hesitant and not sure what to do, they motioned for me to keep going.

I felt like I had just accepted a dare for the team in a game of truth or dare.

Looking back at my teammates, I hoped for some kind of

reassurance or for some sign that beckoned me, and us, to stop. But there was neither. They, too, were not sure what to do.

When I was within five feet of the fence, I stopped. I had no idea what to do. I had no clue what the respectful and appropriate custom might be. The guides once again offered no suggestions. My heart was beating so fast that it was hard to think. And yet, there was a part of me that was trying hard to look confident and fearless not only to my team, but to the villagers who were watching.

What if this community was like the one who stopped us earlier and surrounded our SUV? What if we were unknowingly being impolite or were encroaching on land where we were not welcomed?

Suddenly an arm emerged through the vines and abruptly flung the vines off to the left side, only for the vines to quickly fall back into place. The arm then re-emerged and this time, firmly held back the opening. The arm was strong and immaculately toned, defined with musculature so perfect it was human art.

I quietly gasped as a man stepped forward. Perhaps in his fifties, his face and body were marked with red paint, and through his nose . . . a four-inch-long bone. His eyes were intense, his facial expression stern as he looked at me, then at each member of the team . . . and finally at our guides.

He turned back to me and without blinking, confidently and forcefully spoke. But I did not understand. I turned to Sabby, but the only thing he offered was a shrug. No one was able to understand the language. This was not surprising as more than eight hundred languages are spoken in the country.

I forced a smile and said: *"apinum"* which was 'hello' or 'good afternoon' in the most recent dialect of Tok Pisin that we had learned. There was no warmth in his eyes and no smile. His body language, much like his arms, communicated strength and firmness.

Chapter Eight

Once again, he spoke. Louder and more forceful.

I held my breath as my heart beat faster, thinking he was getting frustrated by my lack of understanding. He then let go of the vines and they fell back into place. At that point, I wondered if we should simply apologize for the intrusion, offer a gift and leave.

Before I could finish the thought process, there was more movement on the other side and I glimpsed through the drapes others gathering only a few feet away, behind the curtain. Moments later, clashing sounds began as sticks protruded through the curtain, moving the vines side to side causing the drapes to swing and undulate. Accompanying the movement were grunting and grumbling sounds much like those of growling animals.

Suddenly another man slung back the vines and stepped forward. His head was covered by thick, black animal hair that hung in front of his face and extended to his jaw bone. The hair was very black, coarse and straight and fit the top of his head snugly, like a toupee. His eyes were hidden beneath the hair, which hung in front of them, and only became visible for brief moments when he turned his head. His demeanor, however, was friendlier than that of the first man.

Without saying a word, he began to scan our group, pausing briefly on each subject as if he was performing a thorough inspection. We remained silent.

A third man, with red facial paintings like the first man, then came to the entrance and stood to his left. He spoke and I once again responded *"apinum."* He then methodically turned and looked at each of us, assessing us as if perhaps to determine if we were trustworthy or if we posed a threat. After a few minutes, he pulled back the opening and with a nod of his head, he invited us to enter.

We remained speechless as they led us to a cleared area, seventy-five feet away. The area was smooth, flat and about the size of half a football field. There was no grass, vegetation or rocks. Surrounding the clearing were several large huts and beyond them . . . the dense jungle.

As we walked, the children and other members of the village began to trickle in behind us. The men who invited us in then joined seven other older men and women in the center of the cleared area. Their attire was spectacular—hues of color that would have made any artist long to capture them on canvas. The faces of several men were painted with numerous parallel red lines across the cheeks and forehead, while shorter perpendicular red lines were drawn from the lower lip to the chin.

Feathers, sticks and plants intertwined with clothing and served as objects for body piercings, especially through the nose, for both men and women.

Most of the women had large rectangular capes, but unlike capes associated with super heroes, these covered their heads and backs and extended down to the backs of their legs. Three to four feet in length and two feet wide, they appeared to be made from the soft inner linings of tree bark.

Two of the women had large clumps of earth with moss on the top of their heads. Long, green sporophytes jutted out from the moss and dangled in front of their faces. Other women had loosely bound bundles of long, slender green leaves that wrapped around their shoulders and hung on the outside of their capes.

Multi-layered strings of shells and bamboo-like wooden pieces crafted elaborate necklaces, which fit around the women's necks and fell softly against their chests while dried grass skirts swished with their every movement. Their faces had various markings of

Chapter Eight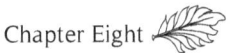

yellow and white, and in their hands, they carried eight-foot-long sticks that looked much like walking sticks. At the top of each stick, a cluster of pink flowers was bound.

The men carried clubs and wooden bows and arrows. In the center of the group was one older man who appeared to be the eldest member and the chief. On his head, he balanced a three-to-four-foot totem that he held with both hands. It was an extraordinary piece of sacred art, an extraordinary display of feathers from the magnificently colored blue birds of paradise, parrots, and a multitude of other exotic birds. Interspersed within the feathers were the tails of possums. Sunlight seemed to hit the totem perfectly as the headdress radiated with every conceivable color. Various shades of blue, red, yellow, orange and green with streaks of white and flashes of brown and black.

Without a word, the chief began to sing and dance, and the others immediately followed. Dancing clockwise in a circle, they moved methodically and slowly. The women's feet glided along the ground, almost like doing the two-step in slow motion. The men both walked and jumped inches above the ground as they moved forward in a processional circle.

Perhaps because I was the leader of our group, I was encouraged to join in and reluctantly did so. The moment I did, the kids started cheering and laughing, and it was not long before the adults were laughing too. At one point, a lady tucked two stems of pink flowers underneath the sides of my bandana. The flowers dangled in front of my face, slightly covering both eyes and gently flapping against my skin each time I jumped up and down. As I made it around the circle each time and got closer to the children, I pulled back the flowers that were in front of my eyes and made a surprise face or danced a little more, which made them scream with excitement.

The dancing and singing eventually slowed and came to a stop. And we were officially welcomed into the village. The chief smiled and motioned for us to come to him.

During the dancing and singing, our guide Sabby had left in search of a translator. He had been told that someone in the village could translate the language of the village to a language he understood, which could then be translated to English. With the translator by his side, Sabby joined us next to the chief, who gave his permission to have a conversation.

After a moment's silence, Sabby nodded to me as if nudging me to start the dialogue. I thanked the chief and his village for allowing us to visit, stating that we were honored to be in his presence and that of his people. As respectfully as I could, I inquired about the beautiful totem that he carried upon his head. Smiling, he said the totem was a symbol of welcoming. He carried it as an invitation for us to enter the village.

With his permission, the team filmed as I walked over to the men and women to look closer at their attire and the plants and bones pierced through their septa. At first, we walked closer to the women who had masses of earth and moss on their heads, but then I was drawn to one particular lady who had a huge cluster of green, leafy stalks protruding through her nose. The bundle looked to be an inch in diameter and six inches in length. I could not fathom how she could breathe through her nose or have a full field of sight. At my intrigue, she smiled, and through the translators, I asked if it hurt or if it itched. With a big grin, she shook her head no and proudly turned to the others who surrounded her.

Chapter Eight

Asking if they kept the piercings in their noses all the time, the chief replied that they did. I then asked him about the smoked bodies that we had heard so much about. The mummies.

He explained that they smoke the bodies of their warriors. After a warrior dies and after a time of mourning, the body is ceremoniously taken to a hut and elevated above a fire where it is smoked for up to a month or longer. They then wrap the body in cloth bandages and coat the outer layer with an orange-red clay to help preserve it. Positioning the skeleton as if it is sitting in a chair, the body is then carefully carried to a ledge high along the mountainside where it remains, protecting the village and land below.

As soon as the translation was completed, the singing and dancing resumed. The conversation was over.

After ten minutes of dancing, the chief slowed and stopped, while the others did likewise. He then pointed toward the top of the mountain to our right, and without a word, several men and young boys started to walk in its direction. We were motioned to follow.

Although I had physically trained for the trek, the climb up the mountain was difficult. In places, the incline was so steep that we had to pull ourselves up by the roots and limbs of trees. Several times we stopped to catch our breath, glancing down at the village below, which was becoming more and more difficult to see.

Arriving at the top, I took several deep breaths and stared at the mummies in front of us. The five-foot-deep, forty-foot-wide ledge, with its exposed wall of dirt and rock, appeared to have been slowly chiseled out of the side of the mountain.

And the Silent Spoke

In front of the mummies, near the cliff's edge, was a slanted, narrow dirt path, one to two feet wide except in the middle section where it diminished to only a few inches. Its slope was steep and its path uneven, demanding that attention be given to every step.

The mummies sat as powerful CEOs, their forearms propped up to shoulder level as if resting on the raised arms of chairs. They sat side by side, facing out over the jungle and village below.

Some of the bodies were bound by one-half-inch to one-inch-wide bandages, made perhaps from the inner bark of trees. Some were coated in orange-red clay while others had only the off-white colored bandages. Still others had no bandages at all. A few of the warriors had been placed in v-shaped wooden structures that served much like baskets, keeping the skeletons intact.

Many of the bodies had fallen apart over time, which resulted in small piles of bones and the fragments of bones on the ground directly in front of the makeshift chairs. Other remnants of skeletons: ribs, femurs, phalanges, skulls . . . were placed in open-faced, three-foot-long wooden coffins which lay on the ground in front of the mummies.

Flies were everywhere, constantly reminding me of the various stages of decomposing, decaying flesh. Darting in and out of eye sockets, nasal and oral cavities, the flies were on tarsals and metatarsals, carpals and metacarpals, ribs and sternums. They navigated the most recently deceased as well as those much older.

It was quiet. Just the breeze and the buzzing of flies. No one spoke. Even the villagers who had accompanied us remained silent as they sat and watched our every move.

A butterfly appeared and landed delicately on one of the skeletons, right where the heart would have been located. I stared in amazement, thinking how the butterfly had often been regarded as a

Chapter Eight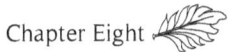

symbol of metamorphosis and rebirth. And of all the places for it to have rested . . . but upon the site of the warrior's once beating heart.

It would be the only butterfly any of us saw that day.

As we continued to observe the smoked bodies, one of the men from the village addressed our guide. He was a young man in his early twenties, and he wore a yellow shirt and brown shorts. Standing up, he proudly pointed to one of the most recently deceased warriors, who was fully intact and coated in a layer of rich, deep orange clay. The young man smiled, claiming the warrior as his grandfather.

I slowly began to understand the connection, reverence and honor given to the warriors by the people in the village. There was immense pride in their heritage and an unbroken bond that connected the living to those beyond.

I sighed. My emotions were mixed as I imagined such a loved one before me. I thought of my own family . . . my grandfathers . . . for they too had passed. With my grandfathers' funerals, there had been an element of finality and closure. Even though I believed that their souls would live forever, my belief was that they would do so in a different realm, not within a specific geographical area.

But in Menyamya, the deceased warriors continued to be an important part of the community. For the KukuKuku people, it was not only the shells of their warrior's physical bodies that remained in the village, but also their souls.

How peaceful it must have been for the warriors at their moments of death to believe that they would continue to protect their families, children, grandchildren and village. Strangely, I also felt protected.

I looked over at the young man whose grandfather sat before us and at the others from the tribe who had accompanied us, who were sitting off to the side of the cliff. For them to allow a group of strangers to visit and to film such a sacred place was a gift. I quietly prayed that others who would come after us would also honor and respect the community and their hallowed traditions.

I sat in front of the mummies and, like them, peered out over the land. It was solemn and peaceful. I soaked up the expansive view of the jungle below, which seemed to go on for thousands of miles. It looked like one continuous gigantic green entity, almost impossible to see any separations or divisions within the matrix. The networks and connections of trees, plants and living organisms within it, however, were undeniably vast.

I thought of the village below. Plants had been uprooted and feathers had been plucked to empower, enliven and decorate the human body, while breathless human bodies adorned the mountainside.

Time and distance morphed as life expanded into dimensions unknown. Dimensions where everything is connected, and everything becomes an integral part of all that was and all that is.

Every day, life was birthed.

And every day, life was extinguished.

And somewhere in-between . . . was I.

Chapter Nine

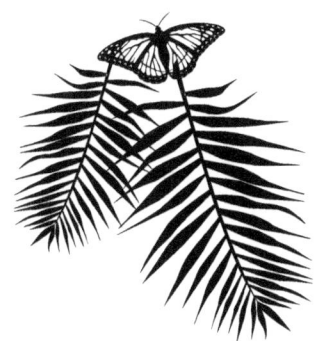

Leaving Menyamya, we traveled the same route back east to Lae. Fortunately, passing through the village where we had previously been stopped was uneventful. It was as though our transit was now insignificant. The sun was shining, and the mud had dried, allowing us to enjoy the beauty and grandeur of the mountain pass and the land without worry.

From the city of Lae we ventured to the northern coast. The original plan had been to take a small plane northwest, to an island that was said to be a favorite of the great oceanographer Jacques Cousteau. I had heard that the island's ocean life and diversity was pristine, and I could only fathom its magnificence, being so beloved to one of the world's greatest ocean explorers.

But two months before leaving the United States, I received an email from our guide, Justin, alerting me that the five-thousand-dollar private plane ride had suddenly jumped to twenty-five thousand dollars. Each way.

The pilot, he explained, had become fearful because of a recent mishap with another pilot who crashed while attempting to land on a small island off the southern coast. Since the island we wished to explore had no airstrip and was very similar to the island on which the other pilot had wrecked, he was afraid that the trip would severely damage or even destroy his plane. Or worse, that it would hurt or kill one or more of us.

With a limited budget, I sought the next best thing—another island not far from it, accessible by boat. Days later, Justin sent an email describing several possible locations to explore, but only one piqued my interest. There was little information about the rarely visited island other than its inhabitants were primarily fisherman who had little interactions with the outside world. The ocean surrounding the island was said to be thriving with life and its coral, unsullied by natural or manmade pollutants.

After arriving in northern Morobe's coastal region, it took two days for Justin to find a boat driver who knew of the island's location. Because there were no commercial materials coming from the island or any trading with the people there, the island had remained mostly unknown.

Few of the boat drivers and owners had even heard of the island, and those who had had no idea of its exact location. Eventually though, Justin found one boat owner who confidently professed that he knew the island and its location, even though he had never been.

The boat driver recommended leaving early in the morning to reach the island by the latter part of the day. Unfortunately, power outages throughout the night had created extensive delays with downloading footage and re-charging batteries. At eight o'clock we were only a fraction of the way through with the downloads and charging. Instead of departing the motel that morning at seven o'clock, we left a little after nine o'clock. With a loaded SUV, we traveled for several hours before meeting our boat driver at the boat's departure point along the shore of the Bismarck Sea.

Chapter Nine

Like a cleared dirt soccer field crammed with people, the boat area looked more like a busy market than any kind of marina. Trash was everywhere. Paper, plastic and aluminum cans were partially embedded in dry dirt, while smaller pieces of plastic and paper flittered randomly with the wind. Along the water's edge, pulled up onto dry land, were dugout canoes and small boats with outboard motors. Gathered around them were small clusters of men and young boys.

Our driver crept at a couple of miles per hour, cautiously moving through the crowd as people walked in front of the moving vehicle as if it was not there. Around the area's perimeter, on the north and east sides, were numerous make-shift stands, swaying slightly in the wind. Beneath the stands' coverings of natural debris and plastic stood merchants selling clothing, food and warm cans of soda.

Ahead of us, a man in the crowd waved and motioned us toward him. Justin announced that he was our boat driver and his name was Rae. When we were within fifteen feet of the water's edge, our driver stopped the SUV. Before we could open the door, Rae was standing a foot away with an outstretched hand.

A young man in his twenties, Rae wore a torn pair of red Nike shorts and a faded blue t-shirt. After initial greetings, he turned and grabbed a large dry bag and, barefoot, led us to his boat. Pausing before stepping inside the boat, he turned around, smiled and said *"plis,"* meaning 'please.'

The thirteen-foot aluminum skiff was a shell of a boat and barely large enough to accommodate our bags, generator, fuel, and the nine of us. Pulling Justin aside, Eduardo, Felix and I discussed our concern for its size, fearing our combined weight would greatly exceed any safe standard, especially with the waves and venturing out to sea. Justin, however, insisted that the boat was more than sufficient and pulled Rae over to reinforce the point.

We piled the bags and equipment high in the center of the boat. Around the mound, each of us found a space in which to squeeze in. Our feet and legs overlapped and intertwined with one another and with the bags. Like awkward pieces of a jigsaw puzzle, everyone and everything somehow fit.

Rae sat beside the outboard motor, pulling the cord several times before it finally started. Quickly giving it full throttle, he surged the boat ahead. The speed caused us to go slightly airborne as the bottom of the boat topped each wave before slamming hard into the sea. Over and over again. While the boat continued to pound the water, Rae jerked the vessel sharply to the left and then to the right before yanking it back to the left and then to the right again . . . playing with the waves. Sitting beside Rae was his assistant, a young man in his early twenties. As his assistant giggled, Rae laughed as if he were a child playing with a new toy. The more air he caught . . . the harder the boat slammed. The sharper the turns . . . the crazier the ride. And the more fun they had.

We, however, were miserable. Including Justin. Our bodies were thrown side to side, knocking into each other and into the bags around us. We sat on the bottom of the boat with no cushioning or padding between our buttocks and the hard aluminum hull, forcing us to take the pounding directly. Shifting our weight from one buttock to the other provided only temporary relief. Although no one complained, we vacillated between laughing and softly moaning.

The possibility that someone might injure their back or break a vertebrae or tailbone was very real. To add to the uneasiness, several of us were becoming nauseated with motion sickness. I was

Chapter Nine

additionally concerned about the added stress on Alec, who had been battling fatigue and a low-grade fever for several days.

Something had to be done to ease the trip for Alec and for all of us. So, without saying a word to the team, I leaned toward Justin and told him that either Rae calm down or he was to turn the boat around, and we would find another boat and driver.

Immediately, Rae slowed the engine, and with its deceleration, the intensity of the pounding lessened dramatically. He also stopped the brash jerking from side to side, which made the ride easier to stomach.

The team sighed with relief.

Rae had estimated that the trip would take five hours. As we neared the five-hour mark, the team became excited with a renewed energy. We could not wait to get out of the boat and to be on solid ground. We could not wait to give our buttocks a rest. And to relieve our bladders.

The five-hour mark came and went.

After six hours we had yet to spot the island.

After seven hours, the island remained out of sight.

We searched hard for the island, but time after time, the land masses we spotted turned out to be nothing more than tiny, uninhabited pieces of earth, dotted with a handful of trees—much like the numerous other islands we had passed during the day.

Not only had Rae miscalculated the amount of time it would take to get to the island, he had horribly erred in its location. I began to question if he had been honest and actually knew where the island was located. I feared also that he was lost and had no idea where we were.

As the day grew late and the light began to fade, our chances of reaching the island before dark became slim. The chatter amongst

Justin, Rae and his assistant escalated as they spoke a dialect of Tok Pisin. When the talking stopped, Justin turned to me and explained that we had to get off the water soon or there would likely be a mishap. Our small skiff had no lights or navigation system, and because there were so many tiny islands, it was impossible to navigate the waters in the darkness without running aground or capsizing. We had no choice but to stop somewhere overnight.

Since our departure, we had passed a few villages when we were navigating closer to the shoreline of the mainland. But no one in our group knew any of the people in the region or anything about them. The thought of stopping at an unknown village, uninvited, made the guides very nervous. To squat on someone's land without permission was not only disrespectful—it was dangerous.

In Papua New Guinea, there are more than one thousand tribes with more than eight hundred languages. From what we were told, deadly tribal disputes were common and mistrust amongst tribes appeared to be the norm. Outsiders, like us, brought another range of complex emotions as we spoke a different language, had a different skin color and were completely unknown.

I worried, and I even thought about the stories we'd heard about cannibalism, although it was rarely discussed. Just the week prior, a tribal elder near the village of Menyamya had shared with us that his father and grandfather had eaten members of warring tribes. When I asked if he also consumed, he quietly denied it.

My gut said otherwise.

Regardless, there was no other choice but to find a village and ask permission to stay overnight.

Chapter Nine

Rae turned the boat southwest, in the direction of the jutting coastline of the mainland and gave the engine full throttle in hopes of finding a sign of village life. After a little over an hour, Rae spotted a faint flickering of light in the distance. Traveling toward the light, it soon became apparent that the light was a fire, and surrounding the fire were the shadowed figures of villagers. As we neared the shore, Rae slowed the engine and steered the boat straight at them.

The approach of our skiff attracted several more villagers, who emerged from the interior and walked to the water's edge. It was difficult to see their faces, but there were men, women and quite a few children. When we were about fifty yards out, Rae turned off the motor, drifting us toward the land. Justin stood and offered a greeting in a local dialect. I was caught off guard by how gingerly he projected his voice . . . soft and hesitant, timid and weak. It was in great contrast to his somewhat pushy, arrogant demeanor, to which we had become accustomed.

A man on the shore quickly responded with the same greeting as more people continued to gather around him. Justin then asked permission for us to come ashore to rest overnight. At Justin's request, a group of men immediately separated from the others and formed a small circle fifty feet to the left of the fire. It was difficult to tell their ages, but they walked more like older men than those of youth. After a few minutes, one man left the circle and walked slowly to the edge of the water. And welcomed us.

As Rae grounded the boat on shore, the villagers smiled, and the kids ran wild. Even though we were in unknown territory, there was something very peaceful about the place.

But just as I was getting out of the boat, Justin grabbed my arm, leaned over and whispered, "We don't trust these people. We may not be safe. Tell your team to stay close."

His words sent a jolt of fear throughout my body.

It was difficult to see the size and extent of the village even with headlamps. While we continued to unload the boat and place our bags on the shore, one of the village elders announced that a family had offered their hut for us to stay in overnight. Not far from our boat, the hut was located in the midst of a group of trees, near the water's edge. With a thatched roof, the fifteen-by-twenty-foot wooden structure was raised five feet off the ground. Inside were two rooms partially separated by a bamboo-like wall.

Thirty feet from it was another hut, and in front of it, three older women squatted next to a fire tending several pots. Behind them was a wooden platform raised two feet off the ground, on which an infant and two toddlers slept. On the ground beneath the children laid a large snoring pig.

Throughout the day, Alec's condition had continued to worsen. Although we believed that it was not contagious, but directly related to his lack of sleep and stress from taking college final exams days before we left the U.S., we made sure to keep him away from the villagers. His fatigue had escalated to a state of exhaustion, coupled with fever and chills. He was so weak that he had difficulty walking. Not only was I worried about him, I was scared. Had his weakened state allowed him to get dengue fever? Malaria? Or some unknown infection?

We prepared his sleeping pad before doing anything else, and he quickly drifted off to sleep. Our videographer, Eduardo, a medic, wilderness survival expert and NOLS instructor, was also worried. The two of us debated the course of action, whether to start medications and, if so, which ones? An antibiotic, an anti-viral or perhaps an anti-malarial? Should we return to Lae and seek the advice of a doctor or medical personnel? Or should we use the satellite phone to seek advice from my physician in the United States?

Chapter Nine

Going back to the hut, Eduardo and I sat on the floor beside Alec, discussing the possible choices with him. Alec, however, declined all options and instead insisted that he only needed to rest. Because there was nothing further we could do, we decided to delay the decision until the morning. While we watched over him as he slept, I silently prayed that the night's rest would do the trick.

With Alec sleeping in the smaller, more ventilated room, we quietly placed the remaining equipment and gear against the walls around him before arranging our sleeping pads in the larger room to his left, just feet away. Alec was resting well, and we did not want to awaken him simply to move him to the other room.

In order for all of us to fit in the room, Simone suggested we position the sleeping pads next to one another, much like the contents of a can of sardines. While we arranged the pads, the two tallest members of our team, Felix and Don, hung the mosquito nets from the wooden planks above.

As we prepared for the night, a soft yell came from outside the hut. At the foot of the stairs stood the elder who had officially welcomed us to the village. Although he did not smile, his disposition was gentle and kind. Moving his left hand toward and then away from his mouth repetitively, he announced, through Justin's translation, that several women were preparing food for us.

It was not long before three women appeared right where the elder had been standing at the bottom of the steps. The first two held out wooden platters of freshly caught and cooked fish with steaming white rice. The third carried a stack of plates and bowls, a conglomeration of different shapes and sizes. Not expecting such hospitality, we were overwhelmed by the kindness and generosity, thanking them in Tok Pisin, the only local language we knew, by saying, *"tenkyo tru."*

After the ladies left, I tossed the protein bars and bags of trail mix we had anticipated eating back into their dry bags and joined the others as we sat and savored the meal. It was moist and flavorful, yet surprisingly not fishy. It was scrumptious.

As we ate, I glanced toward the hut to the right. The three women who had brought the food stood with several others and watched us. Waving to them, I yelled *"tenkyo tru"* and *"namba wan"* meaning 'very good.' The rest of the team quickly did likewise, raving about the food in Tok Pisin and in English. Waving back, the women giggled before carrying on with other activities.

Their generosity was unfathomable. It was well known that rice was not plentiful in such areas, yet they shared their precious supply with us. They had welcomed us even though we were strangers, with different colored skin, a different language and from a foreign land, and even though we had arrived unannounced and uninvited.

As everyone bedded down, there came a beautiful stillness and calm. The hut was forty feet from the water's edge, and the sound of the waves softly crashing against the shore was better than any lullaby. Yet Justin's fear of the village and his words upon our arrival remained foremost in my mind. While the six of us rested comfortably inside the hut, our guides insisted on sleeping just outside the hut's entrance to keep guard.

Because our team consisted not only of members of the 'white clan,' but also of other indigenous Papua New Guinea tribes, Justin was concerned that one or more of us might be considered an enemy and therefore be attacked during the night.

We were no match for the men of the village. We had no means

Chapter Nine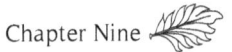

of protection. I continually questioned my decision to go in search of the island and asked myself what I had gotten us into. If anything happened to any member of the team (my friends), I would never be able to forgive myself.

Eventually the team members fell asleep one by one, but I remained awake. Several times during the night I heard the raised voices of men from the village and each time, I held my breath, staying completely still, as if it would help in hearing them more clearly. I'm not sure what good I thought it would do since I was unable to understand a word. Regardless, each time there were voices from the village, there were spontaneous movements and whispers from the guides at the entrance to our hut.

I finally drifted off to sleep in the early hours of the morning, only to be awakened a couple of hours later by a woman starting a fire outside the nearby hut. The night was over, and as I watched her through the only window-like opening in the hut, my worry vanished. She worked diligently, softly humming as she placed small pieces of wood in a central area, one after another. A peacefulness abounded as others in the village began to move and the world awakened.

With the others still asleep and with my newfound serenity, I recalled the long night and felt ashamed for thinking that such a group of people would have harmed us. I wondered if the elders and villagers had greeted the day the same way—relieved that there had not been an incident. Did they also have a restless night of worry because of the strangers who had arrived unexpectedly and uninvited? Had they feared that we would harm their families . . . their women and children? Did they sit up all night in order to protect themselves from *us*?

When we first arrived, I had felt only love and kindness, but then I chose to take on the energy of fear and mistrust as that of our guides, believing that they understood and knew more. However, from the very first moment we saw the villagers from the boat, I believed in the deepest part of my heart that they were good and kind.

I believed too, that we had been divinely led to them and not to another village because they would know that we too were good and kind. I also firmly believed that a higher power had guided and directed all of this for reasons I might never know.

Perhaps though, the experience was to teach me further about the core of human kindness.

After a breakfast of rice and fruit provided by the same women, we spent hours with the elders and the villagers. Alec was feeling much better and joined us as we enjoyed the company of our new friends. We walked through the small village, where several women draped wet clothes over tree limbs for drying, while two young girls spread animal skins across bush-like foliage.

Young boys paddled a small wooden boat in the thirty-foot-wide waterway that ran through the village. The children were between the ages of six and ten and as one paddled, the other two stood and threw spears into the water hoping to pierce fish.

On the outskirts of the village, we met an elder sitting on a tree stump carving a wooden platter into the shape of a fish. In front of him, a pig and her three piglets waddled. Behind him was a hut and near the back of the hut were two young children playing under a tree. The tree seemed to embrace them as its branches leaned close to the ground. Sitting with their legs crossed, they played a game in which they tossed a snail shell into the air, quickly grabbing one or more other snail shells on the ground before catching the one that had been tossed in the air. It was much like the childhood game I played called jacks.

For hours, we walked, talked, laughed and ate together until it was time for us to leave. Before leaving, I told the elders that we hoped to return one day and asked what we might do for them or bring them when we did. I wondered if it might be containers or a system for fresh water, medicine, building materials or even walkie talkies like the ones we had shown them and of which they had become particularly fascinated.

But without hesitation, the chief elder responded, "Education."

Justin translated as he elaborated. "They have heard that children in other villages are being educated. Sometimes, a person will come to the village and teach them. Sometimes, the children travel to become educated. They want their children to have the same opportunities as others. They want them to see the world out there . . . the world beyond their village."

My heart swelled at his response and wisdom. If only I could have captured the response on film for the Healing Seekers' educational materials to share with the schools back in the United States. In the U.S., education is often taken for granted and even regarded as a chore (bordering on punishment) by many children.

Yet here, the elders and the children longed to have such an opportunity. Education was regarded as one of the most privileged gifts in life.

As we loaded the boat and pushed away, the elders and villagers gathered along the water's edge to say good-bye. Motoring away, we waved until we could no longer see one another.

We had arrived at their village after dark, in desperation and need, yet they had welcomed us with open arms. We now departed with their greatest wish and need commissioned in our hearts. And we became determined to do all that we could to fulfill it.

Watching the villagers and the shoreline fade into the distance, I felt a deep sense of gratitude for the unplanned and unexpected encounter. And for the time we shared.

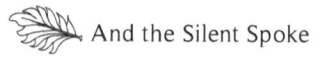 And the Silent Spoke

I began to better understand that there are gifts in life which only arise in moments of vulnerability and helplessness, in moments when we quiet our thoughts and fears. And trust that which is in our hearts.

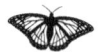

Chapter Ten

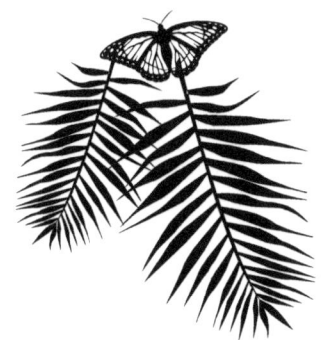

From the village, the island was thought to be another two-hour ride. However, because Rae had underestimated the time it would take to get to the island, he had also miscalculated the amount of gas we would need. Within forty-five minutes of leaving the village, he shut off the motor and emptied the last of several containers of petrol.

Fortunately, before we had left the village, Rae learned from one of the village elders that a man not far away might be able to supply the needed fuel. Carefully steering the boat, he closely followed the coastline as he had been directed until there was a small clearing of trees. Beyond the clearing was a barely visible narrow trail leading into the woods.

Rae grounded the boat, and he and Justin took off down the path while we waited on shore. It took half the day for them to locate the man, purchase and transport the gas. Even with gas in hand, the guides were on edge, as they had no idea if the black-market gas had been mixed with water or if it was even usable. Plus, they had paid a hefty price, closely equivalent to six dollars a gallon.

Regardless, there was no use in worrying. It was the only gas available and it would either work or not. After the containers were loaded into the boat, Rae started the motor and we continued on our way.

Not long thereafter, the remaining gas in the tank ran out. Rae grabbed one of the newly filled containers and poured its contents into the tank before starting it again.

Not one sputter.

The gas was good.

As we neared the island, the seas calmed, and the water became a clear emerald green. The area surrounding the island was like a lagoon, and as the boat moved slowly through its waters, the ocean seemed to be transformed into a massive aquarium filled with the most magnificent fish, sea creatures and coral. Standing up in the boat, we stared at the organisms of bright red, orange, blue, green and yellow that flourished in the world beneath the water's surface. Among them were numerous gigantic royal blue starfish, their plump tentacles spread wide, clinging to surrounding coral.

The reef was breathtaking, appearing as one enormous entity comprised of many variations and moving pieces. Within it were millions of individual organisms. Each playing a part and each contributing to the whole.

Earlier in my life, I had been scuba diving and snorkeling in various tropical areas of the world, but those experiences paled in comparison to the abundant and thriving aquatic ecosystem I was witnessing. The lagoon's underwater world was enchanting and stunningly pure, and it seemed as if I was peering into an endless

Chapter Ten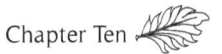

chasm of moving color, with creatures flourishing in a home of fairy tale wonderment.

Our arrival to the island, like our arrival to the village the prior evening, would once again be unannounced. It had never been our intention to be inconsiderate or disrespectful; there were simply no means of communication to ask permission beforehand.

As we neared the island's shore, a man emerged from the tree line and walked to the water's edge. Wearing only a ragged pair of shorts, he smiled and motioned us in.

Rae eased the throttle and gently guided the boat into shallow water. When we were in three feet of water, we jumped over the sides of the boat and exchanged greetings with the man, who was known as Lucas. The moment I set foot on the island, I knew deep within my heart that it had been worth the journey.

Following Lucas, we carried our bags to a small wooden building fifty yards away. With two open, empty rooms, the building served as the village's guesthouse, which was typically used by relatives who were visiting from nearby islands. With our bags inside the two rooms, we went to explore the island with Lucas.

As we walked, and as Justin translated, we shared the interest we had in his island and the hope that we would be allowed time with his medicine man or healer. Eager to oblige, Lucas led us directly to the hut of an elder who often treated the people in the village.

The elder, known as Kupsey, was soft-spoken and shy. And well into his sixties. His beard was predominantly gray and wiry. His hair, the same. While the burgundy T-shirt he wore hung loosely, it was riddled with holes and ripped at the hem.

Kupsey invited us to a small shelter-like hut, located twenty-five yards from his home. Erected a foot above the ground, the shelter had a thatched roof and a wooden floor. Because there were no walls, but only posts to hold up the roof, the ocean breeze flowed freely through it.

In front of the right corner of the shelter was a small fire, and we were asked to sit around it with Kupsey. Conversations took time. The dialect of Tok Pisin that he spoke had to be translated by Justin, while also assuring that the meanings behind the words were correct. Consistently during the conversation, non-verbal gestures were used, such as demonstrating someone throwing up, coughing, or with back pain.

The healer spoke of many things, including his life, family history and his work with plant medicines. He described the days in his youth when he would follow his grandfather near their home on the mainland to find the medicines the older healer needed to treat others. Kupsey explained how he eventually took a boat to this island and made it his home.

Although there were many remedies he used to help those in his village, Kupsey was not known as a medicine man or healer. He was simply a member of the community.

His medical knowledge was not broad, but rather, focused on a few specific issues. There were others in the village, however, who had knowledge of other treatments. It was as if the community had several medical specialists, but not one general practitioner.

Kupsey talked in depth about treatments for malaria and skin conditions. At one point he also spoke of a plant that he used to "help the blood to flow." I wondered if he meant a woman's menstrual cycle, as most cultures have such treatments for women, including special treatments for pregnancies and childbirths.

But it was not for menstrual flow. It was for anyone who had problems with the blood in the body not flowing properly. I asked Kupsey to please help me understand what he meant by "the blood not flowing properly."

Chapter Ten

He stood up and began to describe the problem in both words and gestures. It was if we were playing charades as he mimed and spoke a language I did not understand. Facing me, he let his left arm go limp, hanging loosely by his side. With his left eye slightly closed, he torqued his mouth so that the left side of his face drooped. He then walked, dragging his left leg as if there was paralysis. Even without words, I understood. After he had finished, Justin translated; it was exactly what I had thought.

My heart pounded with excitement as I sat in astonishment. With no formal education, Kupsey described in great detail a person having a stroke. Not only was he describing the symptoms, he was explaining the blood flow and how it was being blocked. The plant, he explained, would help the blood to flow again.

I wondered how he knew of such a plant and how he gained his understanding. I tried to recall the lectures in college where professors had discussed in great detail the process of a blood clot. Terms like thrombi, aggregated platelets, red blood cells and fibrin came rushing back to mind, as did emboli and deep vein thrombosis, tissue factors, coagulation, INRs and fibrinogen.

Advances in Western medicine help monitor, scan, analyze, diagnose and correct issues on multiple levels; however, there were no such methods, laboratory devices or technical equipment on Kupsey's island. Or anywhere near it.

Over the next few days, we continued to learn about the plants Kupsey and other villagers used for medicine while we filmed many aspects of the village's daily life. Children played a form of soccer, kicking an irregularly shaped ball made from pieces of plastic that had been tightly bound. Women sat on the ground under the shade of trees weaving strands of grass into mats. Men and young boys mended fishing nets while others cast nets into shallow waters between waves in hopes of catching fish.

Hiking to the other side of the island, we found ourselves nestled in a magical forest. Above us, a tree canopy of centuries-old hardwoods sheltered the fields of large green ferns below. Trickling water flowed within a small stream, softly rippling over a cascade of tiny waterfalls. Groundcover of bright green moss consumed the land and rocks on either side of the stream, sheltered by ferns and other lush foliage which draped over the water's banks. Birds and butterflies, which I had rarely noticed since our arrival, appeared to flourish.

Lucas explained that the area had remained pristine because the land was sacred. No one was allowed to build a hut or chop down a tree or plant a garden.

Leaving the sacred area, we continued along a barely visible path until Lucas stopped, squatted and pointed to a small plant. With tiny, dark, slender green leaves, the plant was one that I had noticed throughout the day because it was one that grew along the path and was one that we had walked on numerous times.

Looking up at me, he said, "Cancer."

My eyes widened as I squatted beside him and asked how he knew about cancer. Through the translator, he said that his father-in-law had become very sick, and the community came together and transported him many miles by boat to the nearest missionary clinic on the mainland. His father-in-law stayed at the clinic for several weeks. When he returned to the village, he said that the doctors told him that he had breast cancer. They gave him medicine but said that there was nothing they could do to cure him.

Word spread throughout the village. Hearing of his father-in-law's condition, a man in the village told Lucas about a plant that

Chapter Ten

he thought might help. Following the man's instructions, Lucas helped his father-in-law boil and then strain the leaves of this tiny plant. His father-in-law sipped the medicine as a tea. They also prepared a topical application by steaming the plant's leaves and placing the leaves directly across his chest over the affected area.

Lucas's father-in-law improved until he was able to resume his normal activities. With enthusiasm and vigor.

I thought about the plant and how I had disregarded it when I had stepped on it. It never occurred to me that the plants upon the path on which we walked were so important. There had not been anything remarkable or unusual about its appearance; in fact, it might have even been regarded as a weed.

I wondered how many other plants and species of life have been dismissed or neglected, cast aside like weeds. How many species remained untapped and unknown? How many diseases and conditions could be eradicated with their gifts?

How many unknown species had already reached extinction? How devastating have their disappearances been to mankind and to other life forms that depended upon them?

Discussions with Kupsey and Lucas continued well into the evenings, when many others from the village came to visit outside the guesthouse. We talked and laughed as we shared our lives with one another. Pulling out his laptop, Eduardo played video clips from the day's footage as well as showing photos and videos taken in other parts of the world.

They were captivated by our technology . . . the computers, walkie-talkies and cameras; yet, multiple times we stated that the devices and the things we had paled in comparison to the paradise in which they lived. And I believe they knew it to be true.

On the fourth day, we packed our bags and said good-bye. We hugged one another multiple times realizing that neither group wanted the time to end.

Boarding our skiff, we waved to the group gathered on the shore. As I silently vowed to one day return.

The journey back to Lae included one stop to purchase additional fuel. Landing the boat upon the same shore as before, we went in search of the same man Rae and Justin had met only days earlier. While Rae, Justin, Eduardo, Don and I went inland, the others stayed behind with the boat.

Not far from the petrol supply at the man's hut was the village market. Eduardo, Don and I decided to explore the market while Rae and Justin went to purchase the gas.

The market was bustling. Vendors were aligned in two rows that were fifty yards long. With a ten-by-ten-foot space, each vendor sat on the ground with a piece of cloth spread out before them. On top of the fabric, they presented such merchandise as produce, rice, betel nuts and eggs.

Don ventured outside the market area where he surprisingly met a researcher from Germany. Her pale skin in the crowd of Papua New Guineans, he claimed, had been impossible to miss. She explained that she had been there for three months trying to get local villagers, including on a nearby island, to talk with her. As she described the island and its location, Don realized it was the island we had just departed. Although she never elaborated on her

Chapter Ten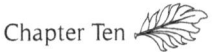

research, it seemed strange such a hospitable village had rejected her request to visit. Several times.

Don explained that we had arrived unannounced but had immediately been welcomed. Speaking of the village's kindness, he shared that we had spent several days with them and that it had been difficult to leave. After verifying once more that it was indeed the same island, Don apologized that his news was likely discouraging to her.

Back at the boat, Don shared the story of his encounter with the scientist with the rest of the team. Speculations surfaced over what might have happened—that maybe the community rejected the kind of research she wanted to do—or possibly, that the community did not feel comfortable with her. We would never know.

Our discussions then turned and focused primarily on gratitude. How blessed we were that the village had accepted and welcomed us. And how grateful we were to not only spend time with them, but for them to become our friends.

During the entire trip, there had been many moments of divine guidance and protection—moments that led to special connections between our group and those we met. In the beginning, on the way to the island, we were in dire need of a place to overnight and had been led to a village that embraced us. The night of good rest had allowed Alec to turn the corner and put him on the path to recovery.

The village also led us to much needed petrol.

Although we had arrived at both villages unannounced, we had been warmly and immediately welcomed. Every encounter had been strongly rooted in some kind of unspoken word and kinship.

Bonds had been formed by the love and energy we shared more so than from the words we spoke or the actions we took.

I'm not sure why the German researcher had not been permitted an audience with the villagers. It is not for me to say. I do believe, however, that there is a purpose for why some things happen and why some do not, and that some things only happen when the time is right. Like the scientist, I, too, have had many experiences in my life where things did not go as I had hoped and planned.

Although my heart ached for her, I realized that during our excursion to the island, everything seemed to be in perfect alignment for our team. For us, it was during those few days that both our timing and our place in the world were impeccable.

God continued to smile upon us, clearing the paths before us while opening our eyes further to the majesty of life. As hearts were opened and deep bonds of friendship were formed, we celebrated our differences as we embraced our oneness.

The island's complex ecosystems remained foremost in my mind. I continued to dwell on the lagoon's unfathomable richness, diversity and expansiveness of life forms, which thrived in such close proximity to each other.

And I thought to myself . . . if millions of organisms can co-exist and thrive together, surely there is a place where humanity, too, can find greater peace on common ground.

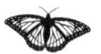

Chapter Eleven

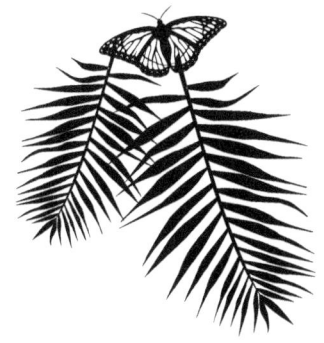

She stopped.
Suddenly, a rather loud and irritating noise resonated throughout the room. At first, it startled her, but then she realized it was yet another one of the nieces' or nephews' technological gadgets. Even though she tried, she could not get used to their beeps, chimes and ringtones.

Many years earlier, she had stopped trying to keep up with all the latest devices, cell phone capabilities, voice activations and other gadgets. The devices, however, were like appendages to her nieces and nephews and the younger generations. From the day her nieces and nephews had arrived, she had been bombarded with a variety of sounds day and night.

The noises seemed monotonous, unpleasant and void of melody. How nice it would have been, she wondered, if they were more pleasant and soothing, like notes from a beautiful piece of music or sweet melodies from an angelic voice.

Before the kids were to leave the following day, she hoped that there would be time to share some of her most favorites, like Thomas Newman, Anthony Griffey, Victoria Livengood, Meredith Holladay, Karin Hougaard, Enya and Enigma. Perhaps that evening over a glass or two of wine.

And the Silent Spoke

She hoped that the music she shared might serve as a catalyst to encourage them to explore the vastness of artistic talent in the world. And to do so at a much younger age than she had done.

Regardless of what the evening might hold, she vowed to simply be present. And enjoy every minute with them.

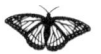

Chapter Twelve

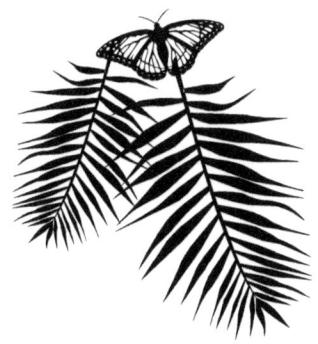

O*nce the noise ceased and the room became quiet once more, she continued.*

With limited days in which to travel and explore, every expedition had to be strategically planned in order to cover as much territory as possible. Throughout Papua New Guinea, we traveled by off-road vehicles, boats and planes. Flights were not always dependable, yet the flights determined our schedule.

For the hours and days surrounding the flights, we created non-stop itineraries in efforts to accomplish all that we possibly could. Our indigenous guides, however, could not grasp the importance we placed on a schedule and on time, which often left us waiting for extended periods. Their lives did not revolve around a clock, nor could they comprehend the need to be so regimented. For them, there was enough time in the day to do all that was needed, and if not, there was always tomorrow.

For our team though, time was invaluable, and the hours spent idle were frustrating. But no matter how many ways and how many times I tried to relay to our guides the importance of keeping to a schedule, time after time we were met with the same outcome.

And so each time, we waited for them to arrive so that we could explore nearby or travel by SUV to our next location. Leaving before dawn allowed an early start to the day. But instead of getting a jump on the day, we sat and waited. Sometimes for hours.

With each occurrence, my frustration mounted further until I became livid at what I felt was a continued disrespect for our team and a lack of appreciation for the expenses we had incurred, which included a premium for the guide service. After exhausting every strategy I could imagine, from kind explanations to lengthy discussions with our main guide, I resorted to using words of the English language that would make my mother wince. Words, which the team later claimed, would have made a sailor blush. Words, too, that I would later regret using in front of others. The team, however, would laugh about it for years.

Regardless, nothing we said or did changed the guides' behavior. Not one of the strategies was effective. And so, we continued to wait each time.

Only twice during the trek do I recall a guide becoming more focused on time than our team. The first was when we were an hour and a half away from the Madang airstrip. While riding in the SUV, our guide Daniel suddenly became anxious and impatient, insisting that the driver hurry.

As we were on schedule, we could not understand his worry. We were slated to arrive in plenty of time to unload our gear and to load the plane. Plus, it was the last flight out that day and small flights were rarely on time. Yet Daniel's restlessness continued and seemed to heighten with every passing minute.

I feared he had not secured our seats on the plane, which had already happened once on the trip. Such a thought made me cringe

Chapter Twelve

because this flight was the critical connection that would get us to Lae and then to Goroka.

Finally arriving at the Madang airport late in the afternoon, Daniel swiftly walked inside the small building to find an attendant. The team, meanwhile, unloaded the SUV, then hauled the bags and equipment through the single door to within a few feet of where Daniel stood in the open room. Leaning up against the counter, he talked to the female attendant on the other side before turning around to us. With a concerned look on his face, he explained that the plane was running behind schedule, but we should go ahead and tag the bags and have them ready to go.

One by one, we placed each bag on a scale to document the weight before placing it on a flat wooden baggage cart that would be used to transfer the bags to the plane. A few feet away from the baggage cart were several hard, white plastic chairs that lined the wall and served as the waiting room.

To the right of the chairs, in the far corner of the room, a young girl stood behind a table tending a small stand. Placing our backpacks in the chairs, we crowded around her and selected a stash of Coca-Cola's, chicken and cheese flavored crackers and several bars of milk chocolate. The snacks were huge treats, even though the milk chocolate was old.

As we each grabbed a seat, enjoying the snacks, Daniel left to make a phone call and to buy betel nut. Like many people in Papua New Guinea, Daniel was addicted to betel nut. Locally known as *buai* (pronounced boo-eye), it was a native cash crop and often referred to as 'green gold.' The practice of chewing betel nut has resulted in Papua New Guinea becoming the country with the highest numbers of oral cancers in the world. Sadly, the chewing practice also extends to small children. Even as young as five years old.

As a stimulant, betel nut heightens energy and increases stamina. According to our driver, Daniel's intake was considerable, so much that it was like consuming six or more cups of strong coffee each day.

Unbeknownst to any of us until then, Daniel had been without betel nut for two days, which I expect felt like an eternity to him. The betel nut's active ingredient is known as arecoline, which is believed to act on the same receptors in the brain as nicotine. I likened Daniel's withdrawal to that of a heavy smoker who had been without a single cigarette for a couple of days.

Daniel habitually chewed twenty to thirty betel nuts a day, maybe more. Depleting his supply sent him into a downward spiral. The withdrawal was harsh on his system and psyche, causing him to become anxious, impatient and depressed until, in the vehicle, his symptoms had further heightened to the point of desperation and panic.

The chewing of betel nut involved mixing together three ingredients: the betel nut, mustard (locally known as *daka*) and lime (locally known as *kambang*). The betel nut itself was about the size of a small egg, green and oval with a texture like that of a lemon.

Thirty minutes after Daniel left, he returned with a new bag of twenty betel nuts, a bag of mustard sticks and a small plastic bag of powdered lime. I walked over to the door and watched him eagerly bite through the outer shell of one of the nuts before peeling it away and popping the inner fibrous seed pod into his mouth. And vigorously chew.

He then grabbed a mustard stick, which looked like a large, roughly textured green bean. Wetting one end of it with his mouth, he then dipped the moistened end into the small plastic bag of lime and swirled the stick, coating it in the slaked powder. And then bit the powdered end off.

Chapter Twelve

Chewing and mixing the three ingredients in his mouth made Daniel's saliva and lips turn bright red. Because swallowing the juice was known to upset the stomach, every minute or two he turned his head to spit.

The red saliva that he expelled on the ground looked like splattered blood. Not only did it look filthy and unsanitary, I wondered about the diseases that could also be spread by his saliva—and the saliva of countless others. Upon the same ground, people walked barefoot, and children crawled.

As Daniel stood outside and chewed, I returned to the others sitting in the wobbly plastic chairs. After an hour, the attendant came over to us to give an update. Relaying a radio message from the pilot, she explained in very broken English that the pilot was running behind schedule and it looked as if he would not be able to fly us out that day.

My anxiety hit the ceiling. It was imperative that we fly out that day. It was the only flight and our only chance to make it to Goroka and to attend the Goroka Festival.

The festival is the largest gathering of indigenous tribes in the country, and it only happens once a year. As the most heterogeneous country in the world, Papua New Guinea is home to a plethora of tribes and cultures, and the Goroka festival allows them to showcase their customs and traditions.

The event had been the primary impetus behind my years of longing to explore Papua New Guinea. The lure had begun with a National Geographic article in which the stunning photos and written content about the festival had immediately been captivating. So enticing was the article that I had carefully torn out the pages of the magazine and tacked them to the bulletin board in the pharmacy. For years, the Goroka article and photos greeted me every time I went into the office, and each time I saw them, I dreamed of the day I would experience the festival and the country.

The thought of missing this celebration of diversity was heart-wrenching. I had planned every detail of the entire expedition around the dates of the festival.

Although I wanted to scream, I kept quiet as the attendant continued to explain the problem with a delayed evening departure.

"English not good. Sorry." She said.

"Flying foxes, um, fly when, um, sun goes down. Plane no fly then," she struggled to relay.

Thinking that we had misunderstood, we questioned, "Flying foxes?"

"Uh huh," she stated as she nodded her head. "Bats. Very big. Bats. Many many. Plane hits. Bad. Very bad."

The more she explained, the better we understood. The flying foxes are gigantic bats, which roost in the thousands. Flying into a colony would be tragic for creatures, plane and occupants.

She continued, telling us that there were strict rules about the end-of-the-day flights. Flying beyond the time limit and disobeying the rules would lead to severe penalties and punishment.

If a person survived to face them.

Dazed, and with a huge sinking feeling in my stomach, I leaned back in my lopsided plastic chair, trying to comprehend what I was hearing. Thousands of bats were threatening to keep us in Madang. And not only for the night, but for days, since it was a Friday and there were no other flights over the weekend. If we did not make the flight that evening, we would miss the entire festival.

There was nothing I could do. There were no other planes . . . anywhere. Traveling by off-road vehicles would have taken too much time, especially since we could not travel after dark because of the dangers of being robbed or held up by bandits.

Chapter Twelve

So, we sat and waited.

And hoped.

And prayed.

As the minutes ticked away, the chances were becoming slim that the plane would make it in time. With every movement of the clock, the dream of seeing the festival began to die. If only I had the power to slow time and to lengthen the seconds and the minutes—moments that were flying by too fast.

A message finally came over the radio, and our team quickly gathered closer to the attendant. Over the radio, the pilot sent word that he was making up lost time in the air and if we could turn it around quickly, he thought that he could make the flight to Goroka. We cheered and eagerly watched for the plane's touchdown.

When it finally arrived, we had thirty minutes to unload the plane, reload and take off. And not one minute more.

Somehow the pilot and attendant made it happen. As the wheels left contact with the airstrip below, according to my watch we had two minutes to spare. I peered out the window looking intently for the bats, which I had hoped to glimpse from a distance, but saw not one.

After a few minutes, I scooted back into my seat, closed my eyes and smiled. We made it.

It was almost ten o'clock in the evening before we landed at the Goroka airstrip. And a little past eleven o'clock before we settled into several rooms at a small hotel. I was so excited about attending the festival the following day that it was almost impossible to sleep. It had been a dream for so long that it was hard to believe that it was now becoming a reality.

The following morning, we were up before sunrise. Grabbing coffee, fruit and bread from the hotel, our team piled into a Toyota Land Cruiser. We were to meet a tribal chief from Mount Hagen at a specific point along the perimeter of the festival. The day prior to our arrival, one of our Goroka guides had met the chief, who then graciously invited our team to be with his village while they prepared for the festival.

Our guide mentioned that it had taken the villagers almost nine hours to travel by foot and then by bus to Goroka from their home in Mount Hagen. Funding for their travel had been very difficult to obtain, especially for the group of twenty. Yet, every year it was a priority of the tribe to attend and to be represented at the festival.

By the time we arrived at the village's gathering area, the sun was beginning to rise. Walking a small dirt path through the woods in the dawn light for almost half an hour, we came upon the members of the tribe. The cleared area in the woods, where they gathered, was quiet and peaceful. Mist from the roofs of two small huts was so thick it looked like smoke, almost as if the huts were on fire.

Some of the members were sitting on the ground while others stood, decorating themselves and one another with colorful cloths and feathers and painting their faces. Seeing us, they stopped briefly and smiled, but then returned to preparing for the festival.

The chief's English name was Michael, and his assistant was Lucy. After exchanging greetings, the chief encouraged us to join in the tribe's ritualistic ceremonial dressings and facial paintings.

Perhaps due to our filming, or maybe because we had connected so well, Michael and Lucy insisted that we become honorary members of their tribe for the festival. Without delay, Lucy began to prep my face for painting the traditional colors and markings.

Chapter Twelve

Taking a small jar of pig grease, she dipped her index and middle fingers inside and pulled out a dollop. She then spread the grease until there was a thin, clear layer all over my face. Although the aroma, which smelled a bit putrid, didn't bother me too much, Lucy found it disgusting. She then stepped to the side to allow a young man to artistically create the tribal design.

In his left hand, the young man cupped a partially folded leaf containing a small amount of ground charcoal, and in his right, he held a stick that looked like a thin wooden painter's brush. Dipping the brush into the charcoal, he carefully drew a large obtuse rectangle with a curved top, one on either side of my face. He then pinched small amounts of the ground charcoal from the leaf with his thumb and forefinger and slowly began to press the charcoal into the pig grease, coloring the areas within the rectangles until they were solid black.

Placing the leaf of charcoal on the ground, he then picked up another leaf that contained a small amount of white paint. While he did so, Lucy explained that the white paint is created by extracting the juice from the bark of a tree, which is later heated and dried before it is mixed with water. As Lucy held a fragment of a broken mirror for me to see my reflection, I watched as the young artist meticulously applied the white paint to the areas beneath the black rectangles, making the lower portions of both cheeks white.

Next, he used yellow paint that Lucy said is created through a process of grinding stone into powder. With the yellow paint, the young man drew an oval around each eye before drawing a continuous yellow line than ran across my eyebrows. Dipping his brush into the yellow paint once more, he drew parallel lines along either side of my nose and then around my lips.

To complete the tribal pattern, he used red paint to color inside the yellow oval rings around my eyes, as well as along the crest of my nose. Lucy then placed a knit hat on my head, seemingly woven from a multitude of odd pieces of fabric with vibrant colors of orange, brown, green and black. Lastly, she strapped a tightly woven band around the knit garment to keep it firmly in place.

Don and Alec also participated in the tribal facial paintings, yet they wore the masculine two-inch-wide solid bands around their heads instead of the hats that the women wore. When everyone was ready, we began the twenty-minute walk to the festival grounds.

As we approached the festival, voices materialized, and the air was filled with song and chant. The tribes were of various sizes, and they gathered one behind the other, forming a line that led to the main entrance to the festival. Leading each group was one or more members who announced their group's presence by lifting high the tribal totem, sign or marker.

Directly in front of us, a group of men chanted. The whites of their eyes were prominent against the bright yellow clay that coated their faces. Necklaces made from the ribs of small mammals aligned perfectly against their chests, much like the white keys of a piano. Around each forehead was tied the dead body of a teal colored tropical bird—with wings spread—cushioned by a band of fluffy red feathers. Behind the band of red feathers was a layer of yellow, red and green flower buds that looked like porcupine quills. And at the crown of each of their heads, rows of large red feathers protruded outward, mixed with the yellow, green, red and blue colors of the flowers of the birds of paradise.

In the group behind us, bodies were covered in dried mud. Their faces were painted black with the exception of a thin, two-inch-long white line drawn underneath their eyes. Narrow headbands were

Chapter Twelve

crafted from strips of soft bark. Fern fronds, held in place by the headbands, jutted out from the top while stringy green vegetation hung down from the headbands, dangling in front of their ears and grazing their shoulders. Necklaces made up of small pieces of bamboo were wrapped around their necks multiple times and were bound so thick that no human flesh was visible. Underneath the bamboo necklaces hung strings of white shells that rested upon their chests.

Every tribe was uniquely different. The gathering created a spectacular display of color—with every conceivable hue seemingly present in the fabrics and ornamental accessories. Ancestral identities were artistically painted on the faces and bodies of members, which were further adorned with headdresses, feathers, shells, masks and skins. Red and white, green and orange, yellow and black, green, white, blue . . . unique and marvelous color combinations and patterns that signified generations of customs and traditions. Gathered together in one place, at one time.

Across the open field, spears and totems rose up and down and were thrust into the air as rattles shook, drums beat, and voices resounded. A twenty-foot-long black snake was hoisted above the heads of several members of one tribe as they danced single file in a swerving pattern, which made the snake's body look as if it was slithering through the air.

Feather sprays interspersed with bare quills, totems crafted with exotic feathers and dead bodies of birds and animals were proudly displayed as human bodies danced barefoot, bending over and standing up, twisting and turning, swirling clockwise and counterclockwise. In almost trancelike states.

Other clans were decorated in moss, clay and leaves, many with strands of shells that were often so heavy and bountiful around their necks that it looked as if they would choke. Grass and fabric skirts worn by both men and women swayed in unison, rhythmically flowing to the beats and chants that filled the air.

Our team spent hours at the festival, mesmerized by the traditional dress, customs and music. To my surprise, several tribes had incorporated Western materials into their attire, including commercial green yarn that was used as a component of one clan's headdress. Another group had replaced the traditional bamboo material used to make its musical instruments with PVC piping.

Before my eyes, I witnessed centuries-old traditions and sacred customs that had survived throughout the generations. And at the same time, I was witnessing the gradual influx of Westernization. I wondered how many tribes would continue to hold fast to their heritage in the years to come. How many would forego their time-honored traditions and instead choose more Western ways?

It had been an honor to witness such a moment in time. The festival was a rare glimpse into history, to a time when man was fully dependent upon the environment and other species, and where man seemed to thrive in nature.

As I thought of the gathering over the next few days, images of the festival flashed in my mind. The faces of men, women and children. One image after another—vibrant colors, designs and accessories—highlighted by remembrances of laughter, music and dance. The festival had been more griping than I had ever dreamed.

I was especially reminded of the facial paintings in the days that followed.

There was only one color of which I had neglected to ask the origin, and it was the one color that failed to wash off. For several days, the areas around my eyes and the crest of my nose remained

Chapter Twelve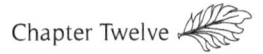

red. With repeated scrubbings, the red eventually faded to pink before completely wearing off.

Michael, Lucy, the Mount Hagen tribe and the Goroka Festival, however, would never fade in my memory . . . or in my heart.

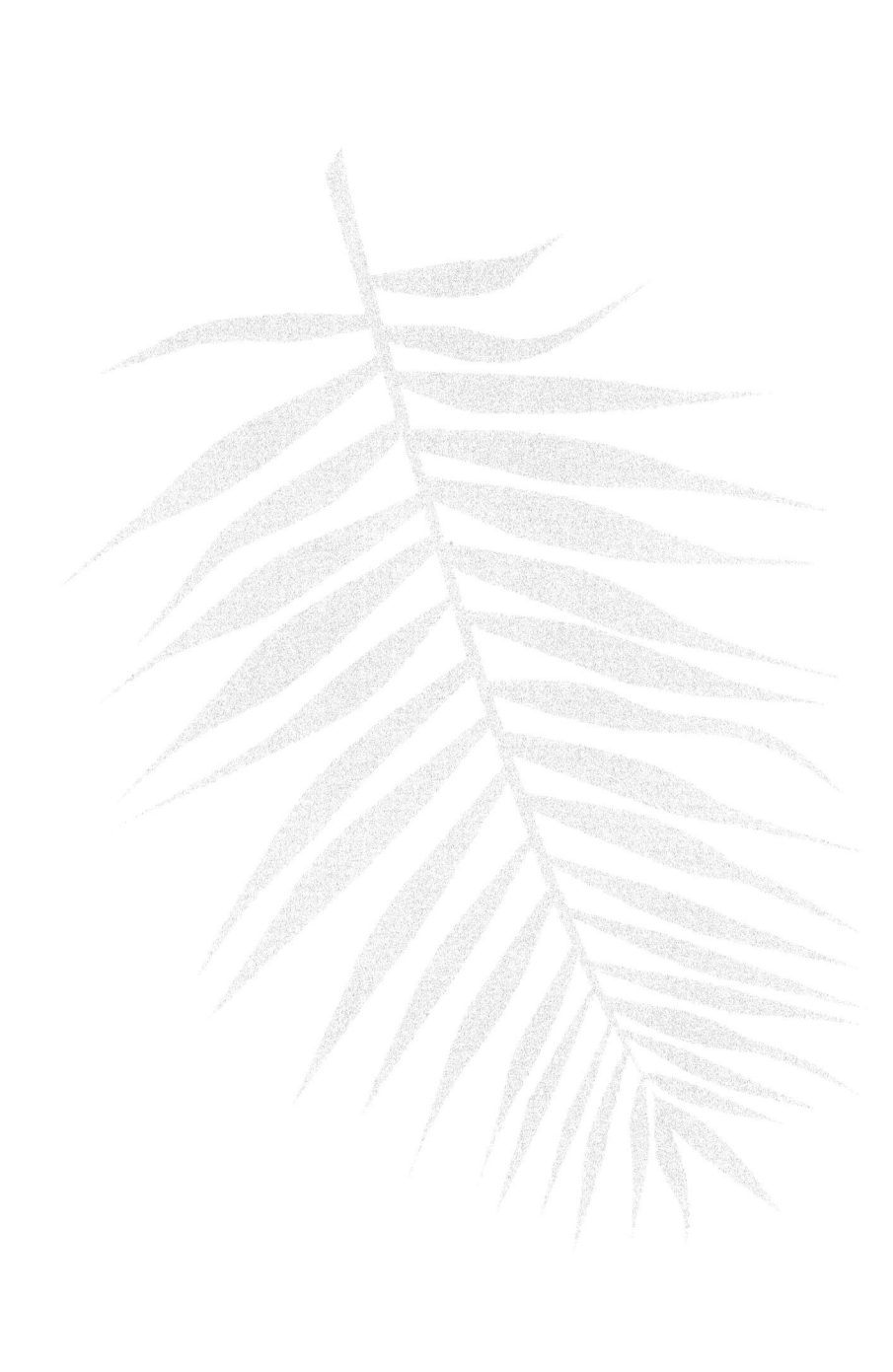

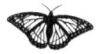

Chapter Thirteen

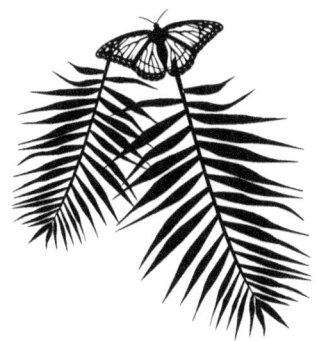

After the Goroka Show, we traveled west along the Highlands Highway to Mount Hagen. Although Michael, Lucy and the tribe lived in Mount Hagen, they remained in Goroka for several more days. We, therefore, were unable to visit with them in their village.

Traveling the Highlands Highway was what I had dreaded most about the entire trek. Armed robberies and attacks along the road are so bad, our driver, Konia, relayed, that the highway is regarded as the most dangerous in the country . . . and one of the most dangerous in the world.

The stretch of highway is notorious for bandits who rob drivers and passengers, and who have been known to rape and kill. Their guns and ammunition, primarily acquired through black market trade, are obtained by bartering with a high-quality strain of marijuana, known as 'Niugini gold.'

The bandits, locally known as *'raskols,'* are particularly active in the more isolated segments of the highway. These areas are often in the mountainous region, where sharp, winding curves prevent the driver and occupants from seeing stretches of road ahead.

Hearing an oncoming vehicle, a raskol gang quickly creates a roadblock by dragging a tree or other large item across the road. This is typically done in a section beyond a blind curve. The unsuspecting driver will come around the corner and slam on the brakes to avoid hitting the barricade. But before the driver can shift the vehicle into reverse to flee in the opposite direction, another group of raskols places a second tree or barrier across the road behind him.

Trapped, the driver, occupants and cargo are at the mercy of the bandits who rob them at gunpoint. Or worse.

In our SUV, we had two hired gunmen from a respectable security agency in Goroka. The agency also provided Konia, our driver. One gunman sat in the front passenger seat and the second, directly behind the driver. Semi-automatic weapons rested on both their laps.

The strategy, according to Konia, was to drive as fast as possible so that the raskols did not have time to act. The road, however, was in disarray, with fractured pavement and large holes that were often several feet wide. This made it impossible to maintain any consistent speed. Konia, therefore, constantly swerved back and forth across the road as he floored the gas pedal only to suddenly slam on the brakes. Accelerating and braking, jerking left to right, back and forth.

Occasionally we encountered a stretch of road that had only limited damage, allowing Konia to accelerate to ninety miles per hour and above. No matter the speed or the haphazard pattern he followed, it was tense and nerve-wracking.

Two hours into the drive, Eduardo asked to stop for a quick "bathroom break." Without taking his eyes off the road or his foot off the accelerator, Konia apologized and said he could not. It was much too dangerous.

We had a little over three hours to go.

Chapter Thirteen

Two hours later, however, Konia unexpectedly pulled off to the side of the road and said that we had three minutes. The gunmen spoke loudly to Konia in Tok Pisin, agitated and upset with the stop. Konia, nonetheless, put the SUV in park while translating that the guards were very concerned because every minute we sat still we became a greater target. Remaining any longer than those few minutes would be too risky.

The gunmen quickly got out of the stopped vehicle. Their guns were held close to their chests; left hands stoically gripping the forends while right hands clinched the pistol grips. Their index fingers extended next to the triggers. One walked briskly along the road in the direction in which we were headed, while the other walked just as rapidly in the direction from which we came.

Since two members of our team had left the week prior in order to return to the United States, I was now the only female. As such, I ran across the road to the closest brush while the guys lined up behind the vehicle.

In the distance, loud voices echoed, yet it was impossible to know if they were friend or foe. Moments later, though, other voices appeared . . . louder and closer, causing the gunmen to turn and jog back toward the vehicle. As they did so, they whistled while moving their left forearms as if they were slowly but firmly chopping the air in front of them, directing us to get back into the vehicle.

Running back across the road, I jumped into the SUV behind the others as the second gunman followed on my heels, breathing down my neck while pressing his hand against my back. Before he could close the door, Konia floored the gas pedal and spun out. Through the back windows, we peered through the dust cloud that formed in our wake . . . but saw no one.

There were brief moments during the drive when I would begin to relax, only to be jarred back into reality with the slamming of brakes and swerving to dodge yet another hole in the road or broken section of pavement. Since raskols were more active at night and the highway much more dangerous after dark, it was imperative that we arrive in Mount Hagen during the daylight hours.

Time, however, moved ever so slowly. The hours dragged and the drive seemed to take forever.

Finally, in the far distance, we saw the city lights of Mount Hagen. As the capital of the Western Highlands Province, it was also the third largest city in Papua New Guinea. And it was our finish line.

Safely in Mount Hagen, I realized how the tension and anxiety of traveling the Highlands Highway had made the hours seem more like days as I had wished for the time to move more swiftly. These feelings about time were in deep contrast to the feelings of angst I had felt days earlier as we waited at the airstrip, fearing that the minutes were passing much too quickly, and the pilot would not arrive in time to fly us to Goroka.

I then imagined what Daniel experienced during the days of his withdrawal as his cravings for betel nut heightened. Yearning for his next fix, he had pressured the driver to go faster as each passing minute, he later confided, felt like an eternity.

No matter the situation, whether it appeared that time was passing by too fast . . . or seemed to stand still . . . time had simply

Chapter Thirteen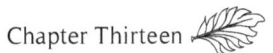

remained constant. Each day had the same number of hours. Each hour, the same number of minutes. Each minute, the same number of seconds.

Time had remained as it always had . . . steadfast and consistent, unwavering and unfaltering.

Even as we pined to prolong it . . . or longed to hasten it.

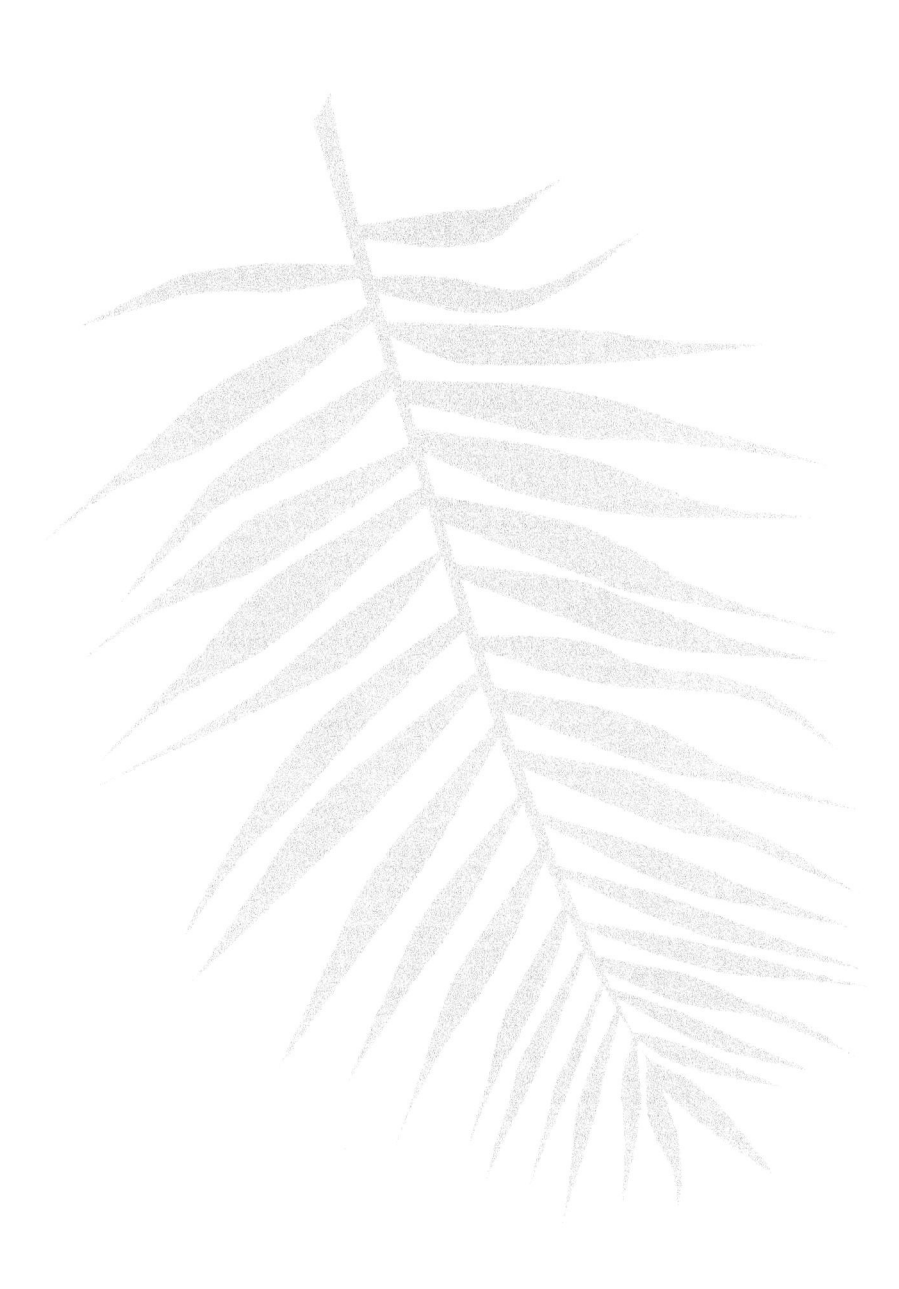

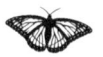

Chapter Fourteen

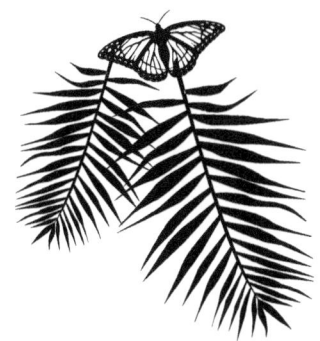

Dominga had prepared a simple lunch. Sandwiches of roast beef, turkey, avocado and the works with a selection of chips, warm brownies and apple fritters. Strangely, though, the room smelled of french fries.

As they ate, conversations flowed with numerous questions and comments about the adventures. While the nieces and nephews discussed the stories and shared their individual perspectives, her mind wondered elsewhere.

She imagined the individuals they might become and pondered the impact they would continue to have upon each others' lives. They had always been close, and in her recollection, she had never heard a harsh or angry word amongst them.

Her mind then drifted to the people they called friends. Were her nieces and nephews aware of the extent to which these friendships were influencing their lives? Did they think about the degree to which these relationships would mold who they would ultimately become?

Silently she prayed that each of her nieces and nephews would be blessed with loyal, meaningful friendships. Friendships that were strong *enough to get through life's trials and tribulations . . . friendships that were based on a love deep enough to withstand the test of time.*

The temperature outside was dropping. A chilling breeze came through a slightly opened window, causing her body to slightly shiver.

Her sensitivity to cold was nothing unusual; she had dealt with it her entire life. Only when she started taking a blood thinner years earlier did her sensitivity become burdensome. The winter months were aggravating, as she found it difficult to stay warm, even when she kept the thermostat at eighty degrees. Frequently, the cold temperatures chilled her to the bone, especially in her right hip due to two hip replacements—creating both discomfort and pain.

Noticing her unease, her nephew grabbed a thick afghan and gently covered her. Then, he kissed her left cheek.

Warm and comfortable, she continued.

Looking back over the years, I now see how my life has been but a tiny thread in the tapestry of life; microscopically woven with all of humanity and all of life. The decisions and actions of others have affected and influenced my life, and my decisions and actions have influenced and affected others.

My connections with others and the world have been varied and complex . . . vast networks and depths of energetic exchanges that I, for my part, have been incapable of comprehending. How is it possible to think of someone whom I haven't seen in months, only to run into them the same day at the grocery store? How is it that I can meet someone for the first time and feel like I've known them my entire life? What is it that lured me to one place over another . . . and to one person over another?

Chapter Fourteen

There was much more to the decisions I made, the actions I took, the feelings I had and the circumstances I encountered than what I could understand or rationalize. There was something much stronger and wiser in control; a divine, intangible force that loved, guided and protected me throughout life.

And it was this divine force that orchestrated my seemingly random connections to people . . . and to places . . . all over the world.

These chance encounters with diverse networks of people and the geographical locations would forever change me. They would teach me that no matter how much I thought I was in control of my life, I was being led, and my hand was being held, by One much greater.

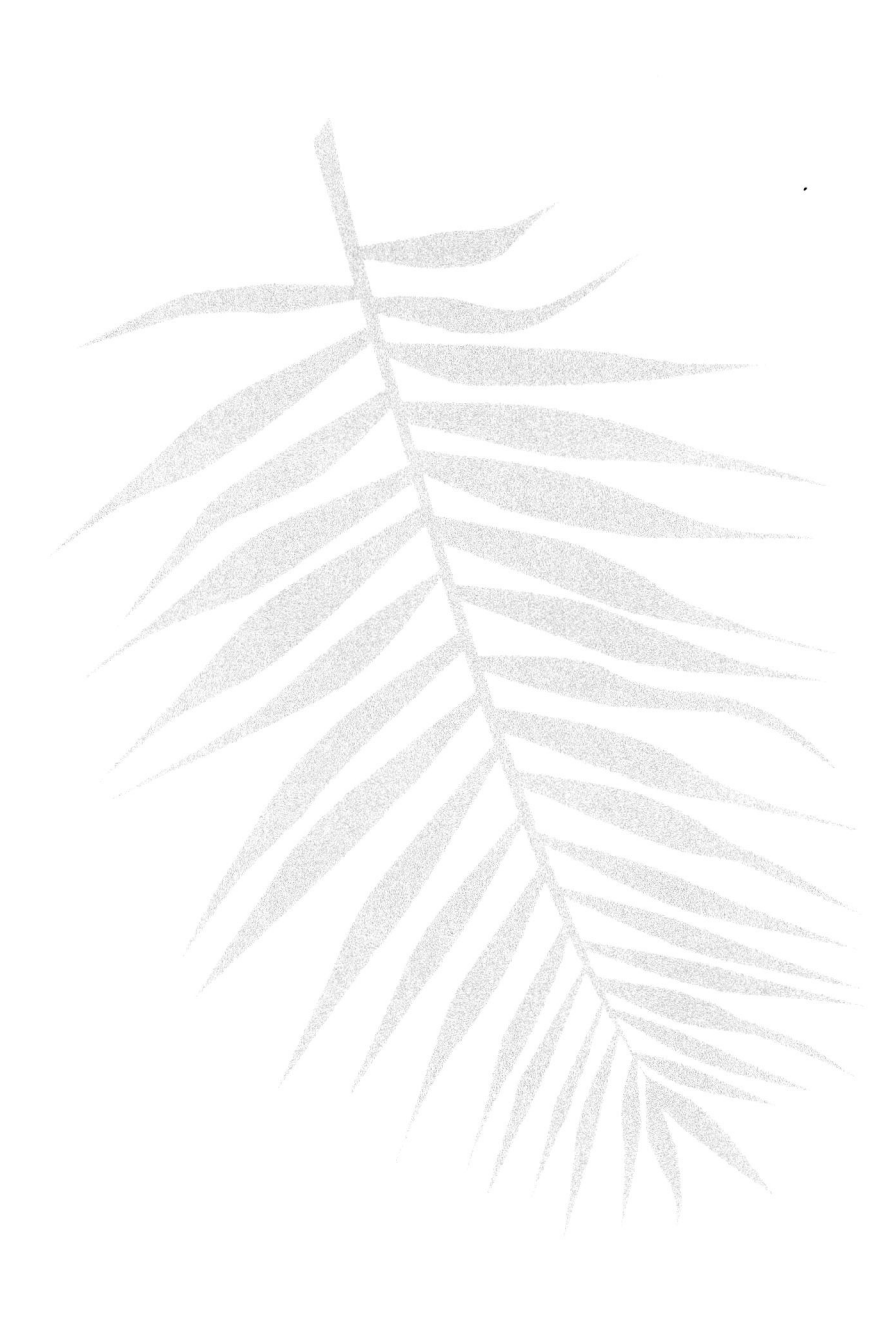

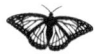

Chapter Fifteen

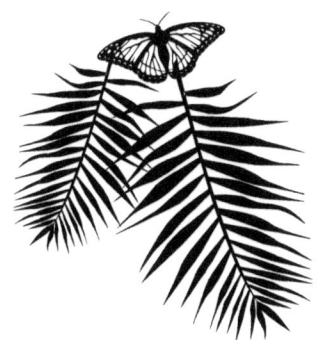

Two years later, we returned to Papua New Guinea. It was mid-September when our six-member team boarded a plane in Lae for the community of Wewak. Because our guide, Justin, had waited until just a few days prior to book the flight, the team was separated and sat scattered near the back of the plane.

As the other twenty or so passengers boarded, I noticed a small group near the front of the plane who appeared to be traveling together. There was little talk as the women took their seats and the men placed items in the overhead bins. There were a couple of coats, a few cloth bags filled with what looked like purchases from their trip and several dried flower arrangements, which they carefully placed at the very top.

The flight was quiet, and we seized the rare opportunity to sleep during the day, even resting during the thirty-minute stopover in Madang when several passengers deplaned. Eventually, the plane landed softly on the Wewak airstrip and with the others, we stepped out of the plane and down the wobbly stairs.

As we walked toward the wooden platform where our bags would be off-loaded, we heard a bizarre and unusual sound. It was a low resonance at first, but the farther we walked away from the plane's engines, the more audible it became. Soon, it was apparent that the murmurings were voices, which seemed to be a combination of crying and wailing, coupled with yells and loud cries similar to those I had heard during tribal ceremonies.

It wasn't long before our team realized that the voices were coming from a group of men and women clustered behind a nearby ten-foot-tall metal fence, which separated the airstrip and passengers from others. The individuals in the crowd numbered close to fifty and ranged in age from teenagers to the very elderly. Those in the very front had their fingers entwined with the chain links, forcefully pushing and pulling, causing the fence to loudly rattle.

Their bellows seemed grief-stricken, yet infuriated and enraged. Their eyes appeared to be upon our group's every move, and as we were the only outsiders anywhere around, I feared the demonstration was against our arrival.

Following the other passengers, we walked to the designated area where we would collect our bags. I couldn't help but stare at the group whose voices seemed to be getting louder by the minute. In particular, my attention was drawn to four young men who had climbed and then straddled the top of the fence, thrusting their fists into the air, perhaps either in anger or in protest. I couldn't say.

Beneath them, standing on the ground, pushing against the fence, women cried uncontrollably. Two of them were so weak that they were being held up by those next to them, while others clasped their hands to their faces as their bodies shook with emotion. Yellow and gray paint marked the faces of both men and women. And were streaked by tears.

Chapter Fifteen

While we, as a group of outsiders, tried to grasp what was going on, our second guide, Winston, walked over and firmly grabbed my arm. Leaning close to my ear, he whispered that we had to leave immediately and insisted that I direct the team to follow. Holding tight to my upper arm, he powered through the crowd waiting at the baggage claim area and headed in the direction opposite of the people at the fence. Closely behind me, the rest of the team followed single file. Behind the team were two men who had quickly grabbed four of our bags off the luggage cart. Above each of their heads, they carried one large dry bag and, on their backs, another.

Winston walked quickly to the back gate of the airstrip where our SUV was waiting. Standing next to the vehicle were two men, who, upon seeing us, opened the back doors and motioned for us to hurry. As soon as we climbed in, the doors were slammed shut. Winston climbed in the front passenger's seat while one of the men got into the driver's seat. The two men carrying the bags, meanwhile, tossed them into the back of the vehicle before going back to retrieve the remaining bags.

Winston turned around. "As soon as we have all the bags, we will leave. Once we were out of the area, I will explain our situation."

I was numb, completely bewildered and yet something deep within told me everything was okay. Even though I didn't really know Winston and had never met the driver or the two men who were collecting the rest of our bags, I trusted that they were protecting us—and keeping us safe.

Within minutes, the two men walked briskly to the back of the SUV, flung open the rear door and plopped the bags on top of the others. Shutting the rear door, they walked around and slung open the side door, jumped in and, pushing several bags aside, sat on the seat directly behind the driver and Winston.

Without a word, Winston and the two men nervously looked around, peering out the front, side and back windows while the driver accelerated and drove away from the airstrip.

Of the four men, Winston was the only one we had met. The driver and the two men who had retrieved our luggage were new to us. It was not unusual, as every new territory required different drivers and guides. What was unusual was not to have introductions immediately. Even more perplexing and strange, however, was that our main guide Justin was missing from our group.

The team members whispered, "Are we in danger? Where is Justin? What's going on?" Typically, I would have insisted on introductions immediately. It was not only a matter of respect and acknowledgement for our new team members, but it also ensured that we knew who were our guides and who were not. It was common that a guide or driver would make money on the side by allowing strangers to ride in hired vehicles. Such passengers often opened the doors to other problems.

But under the current circumstances, the routine—with its introductions—didn't seem to be a priority.

As we pulled away from the airstrip, Winston turned around in his front passenger seat once more and began to explain.

"Unbeknownst to any of us, our plane was transporting the body of a young man who was brutally murdered a few days ago. The family members were sitting near the front of the plane, accompanying the body home."

I sat in silence, remembering the group placing items into the overhead bins. The dried flower arrangements that had been so delicately placed on top of the other items were to adorn the graveside.

"All those people at the fence were members of the family's community," Winston continued. "Gathered to meet the family and form the processional to take the body home.

Chapter Fifteen

They are grieving. The village has lost a member. They have lost a son.

And they are angry."

Winston went on to describe the situation while I tried to process his words. The young man had been killed by a man who was a member of a different tribe. Unless the two tribes made peace or had a quick resolution, it was custom in many areas in Papua New Guinea that the death must be avenged by killing a member of the murderer's clan.

The revenge could be against any member of the murderer's clan, even if the individual had nothing to do with the death. Or had any affiliation to the murderer.

When our plane landed and while our two new guides and driver were waiting on us near the wooden platform, they overheard several people speaking of the death and conflict. When our group deplaned, several men of the deceased man's tribe spotted Justin walking with us, and began asking a lot of questions, trying to verify his tribe. Although the two guides and our driver strongly denied any affiliation, Justin was indeed a member of the murderer's clan.

Justin had been recognized primarily by his prominent facial features. His broad nose and angular jaw line with his deeper, inset brown eyes helped to distinguish his tribal lineage. Fearing that Justin would be attacked and killed, the two guides surrounded him, continuing to deny any tribal affiliation, and whisked him away. During the same time, the driver, Nigel, left to bring the vehicle closer, and to the back part of the airstrip.

According to Winston, for the tribe to have retribution—especially on such a day of deep mourning and heightened emotions—would have briefly lessened their sorrow and diminished their anger. Killing Justin, or any member of the murderer's clan, would have brought a moment of celebration, knowing that the young man's death had quickly been avenged.

Had Justin been spotted on the plane, fighting would have immediately broken out, which could have been disastrous. Despite our awkward seating at the back of the plane, it was fortunate that we had boarded from the rear of the plane while the family had boarded from the front of the plane, thereby keeping Justin out of their direct sight. Had it not been for Justin's last-minute purchase of our tickets, it might have been a different story.

The two guides who had flanked Justin had hidden him in the back of our SUV after safely extricating him from the inquisitive crowd. As I turned to look, the four-foot pile of bags and equipment behind us shifted slightly, and out peeked Justin's head. With his small body hidden between two floppy duffle bags, he nodded slightly and then retreated.

Winston, along with our driver, Nigel, and the two guides became ever vigilant in watching the road behind us, afraid that the men who were inquiring about Justin at the airport would follow. Our fairly new Toyota Land Cruiser was uncommon in the area and therefore easy to spot. And because Justin had been identified with white people, he became an even easier target as we were likely the only outsiders in the area.

Our destination was the Sepik River. Unfortunately, the only road that led to our pick-up point along the river was one that passed through the deceased young man's village. Winston took charge and after discussing with Nigel, decided to forego our scheduled overnight stop, which happened to be in a village that was located near the deceased young man's village. Instead, Nigel would drive nonstop so that we would pass through the family's village late at night. They believed the darkness would give us a greater chance of passing unnoticed.

Chapter Fifteen

I sat in the backseat within an arm's reach of where Justin had squeezed between the yellow North Face and green NRS bags. Every so often, I leaned back and asked if he was okay. From the pile, bags would shuffle, and his hand would emerge, followed by the outline of his face. Each time, he quietly responded, "yes, thank you," before disappearing again.

Other than the times I checked on him, Justin rarely moved during the next four hours. And during the next four hours, other than his brief responses to my questions, he didn't utter a word.

As we neared the deceased young man's village, Nigel, Winston and the other guides squirmed as they spoke to one another in Tok Pisin. Winston relayed to us that they were concerned about a possible roadblock or some other trap for Justin. My fears heightened further when he said that an attack on Justin would also be an attack on all of us.

Eduardo whispered, "Guys, just stay calm. If we have a situation, just stay calm and silent. This is not a time for anyone to try to be a hero."

In broken English, Nigel then spoke of the intense emotions and brutal slayings involved in avenging deaths. He spoke of machetes and guns, spears and rocks. In a stupor, we listened, not wanting to hear his words and yet, not wanting his words to end. With anticipation we awaited the words that would reassure us that everything was going to be okay. But they never came.

As anxious as our team was, it seemed the guides were even more so. In our vehicle, there were only a few machetes. There were no guns, no spears, no means to protect ourselves. Nigel explained that he would drive very fast through the village, and if there was some kind of block in the road, he would do his best to not stop, but drive around it if possible.

I prayed that there were no roadblocks and that we would pass quickly and unnoticed. I also prayed that we didn't hit one of the many deep holes in the road and have a flat tire or other mechanical problem that would force us to pull off to the side.

As we neared the village, Nigel pressed the gas pedal further. Under different circumstances, his driving would have been considered reckless and frightening with his jerking of the steering wheel from left to right and back again, avoiding the holes and broken pavement. But, for us, his confidence and control made us quietly root for him to go even faster.

Reaching the small village, we passed a couple of people walking along the roadside. Twenty to thirty huts lined either side of the road and stretched out over a quarter of a mile. In front of the huts were roaring fires, and around the fires, shadowed figures. No one seemed to care that we were passing though. No one yelled. No one placed a road block.

After passing through the village, we rode for another thirty minutes until Nigel slowed and explained that we would soon stop for the night. The emotional drain had been taxing on everyone. Especially Justin. Nigel knew of a place that was not known by many outside of the area, and felt it would be the safest place for us to rest for a few hours.

It wasn't long before we pulled off the partially paved road onto a narrow dirt road. Moments later, the SUV stopped in front of an old wooden building. With walls that contained rotten boards, the design was much like a motel. Doors were evenly spaced on one side of the building, each leading into individual rooms. Inside each room—a mattress, mosquito net and a bucket of warm, brown water with which to wash.

Chapter Fifteen

Although the structure was off the main road and somewhat hidden, the locals knew it well. According to Winston, word of visitors spread fast in such areas and therefore, it was wise to not remain there any longer than necessary. And though it was rare in Papua New Guinea for someone in a village to own a vehicle due to the tremendous expense, Winston worried that if word of our arrival traveled quickly to the deceased man's village, that they could, with vehicles, reach us before the night was over.

Regardless, Winston felt we should try to get a few hours of sleep and leave early in the morning before daybreak—before anyone else had an opportunity to ask questions or set eyes upon Justin.

Our guides in Papua New Guinea preferred to sleep outdoors or in the vehicles during the few times we stayed in guesthouses or motels so that they could save their pay for other things. That night, however, I insisted on paying for them to stay inside rooms so that they would feel safer and would hopefully rest. Although there were two available rooms for the four of them, they insisted on only using one room so that they could better protect Justin, by surrounding him throughout the night and taking shifts to stay on guard.

Their empathy and altruism toward Justin were astonishing.

We awakened early the next morning without incident. Still edgy and restless though, we packed the vehicle promptly and left. It would take another hour and a half to reach the river.

Spotting the large hardwood tree that marked the designated point of entry to the river, Nigel maneuvered the vehicle off-road through brush and around smaller trees, over dried soil terrain, until he steered it close to the water's edge. And stopped.

The river was pristine, and its flow, swift. Trees and vegetation covered the landscape and hugged its banks for as far as we could see. The dugouts, however, which were to meet us there, were nowhere to be seen.

Anticipating the boats' arrival at any moment, we unloaded the vehicle and stacked the bags and equipment close to the river. Justin, on the other hand, walked a hundred feet inland. He crouched beneath the low-hanging branches of a tree. A few feet away on either side squatted the two guides who continued to serve as bodyguards, intently watching the surrounding area.

Although it took us fifteen minutes to unload and reorganize the gear, the boats that the local guides had arranged remained out of sight. And so we waited.

And waited.

For several hours we waited, and with each passing minute we felt more vulnerable and restless. At one point, Eduardo and I walked along the river bank for about a mile to scout the bends ahead for any signs of the boats, only to return disappointed.

Almost an hour later, Winston whistled. Smiling, he pointed upstream where two long wooden dugouts came into view. As the boats got closer, one of the drivers waved his left hand with a large swooping motion as he continued to manage the outboard motor with his right.

As Winston and Felix pulled the boats partially onto dry land, we loaded the bags and gear, dispersing and balancing the weight with that of the team members. With the exception of our SUV driver, Nigel, everyone would continue with us.

One by one, each person walked down the center toward the back of one of the boats, carefully balancing himself or herself until reaching a spot to settle. Backpacks served as seat cushions while

Chapter Fifteen

our legs served as chair backs for the ones in front of us. With each body squeezed into a small space and with arms resting on the gunwales, Winston whistled to the drivers to move ahead.

Shoving off into deeper water, the boat drivers started the outboard motors and steered upstream. Moving farther away from our departure point, there was a noticeable shift in energy. A happiness filled the air. Team members from both boats laughed and chatted, and with this new energy, the nervousness and anxiety were relinquished.

Justin sat directly in front of me in the first canoe. My knees were up against his back; his shirt gently flapping in the wind. I leaned forward, softly placing my hand on his back and telling him that it was going to be all right. He slowly turned around, looked at me and forced a smile.

As we talked to one another, I began to grasp a deeper insight into what he had experienced during the past few hours.

"I am deeply saddened by the young man's death," he said. "As a father, I cry for the parents. It is impossible for me to think of the heartbreak and the loss they must feel."

Turning his head toward the front of the boat for a moment, as if to gain his composure, he then turned back around and continued, "But, for hours, I feared I would never see my wife and children again. I worried they would never see me again."

Tears formed in his eyes as he looked directly into mine. "I was terrified, but I was also angry. Very angry. This man from my tribe who killed the other, I do not know him. I have never met him. I do not even know his family. Yet, I am the one who could die for his actions."

He continued. "It is the way of Papua New Guinea, Amy. A death must be avenged. Someone must be the sacrifice. Even my wife and children are now in danger as they too are sacrificial candidates.

But if it comes to my wife, my children or me . . . I want it to be me."

Tears welled up in his eyes as they did in mine. Lowering his head, he slowly turned around and faced the expansiveness of the river ahead.

I continued to dwell on Justin and the circumstances surrounding the young man's death for quite some time. I was saddened and also perplexed by the traditional beliefs and customs that had continued for generations, especially knowing that Winston and the other guides, and now Justin, strongly disapproved of the practice.

I wondered if others, especially the members of warring tribes, really wanted to continue the practice of retribution, a practice that involved innocent people—including their own family members. The avenging of deaths from a single event could go on for generations, forcing families and communities to be both predator and prey.

Back and forth.

One life for another.

Men. Women. Children.

Acts of revenge and retaliation like those in Papua New Guinea continue to exist throughout the world. They have been the impetus for conflicts and wars, strife and continued violence. They are carried out in the name of religion, tradition and social, racial and economic circumstances.

Future generations, which are far removed from the initial occurrence or incident, continue to carry the torches of anger, vindication and victimhood of their forefathers. Oppression is battled only to be introduced as another form in future generations . . . thus furthering the cycle of hatred and divisiveness.

Chapter Fifteen

I wondered at what point individuals would be held responsible and accountable for their own actions. At what point would neighbors and friends, children, grandchildren and future generations become free from the actions and sins of their ancestors, groups and communities? Just as Justin was not responsible for the young man's death, neither were his wife and children or their future generations. And nor were the murderer's family and community responsible for the slayer's actions.

As I sat in silence and pondered, the river and the land on either side pulsated with life. It was calm and peaceful. Silently, I prayed that such serenity and tranquility would be brought to the two warring tribes.

I thought of Gandhi, Mother Teresa, Malala Yousafzai and many others in history who challenged the status quo and instigated transformation. Sometimes it only took one person to stand up and say, "enough." One person to become the catalyst for change. One person who was strong enough to lead others and usher in a long-awaited peace.

One person to shift the thinking of a majority.

I prayed for such a person or persons to emerge. For I imagined that when they did, they would discover that they were not alone, that there were a great many others who thought and felt the same way. And even though many had been unable to stand up and speak or intercede . . . they had quietly been longing for another to lead.

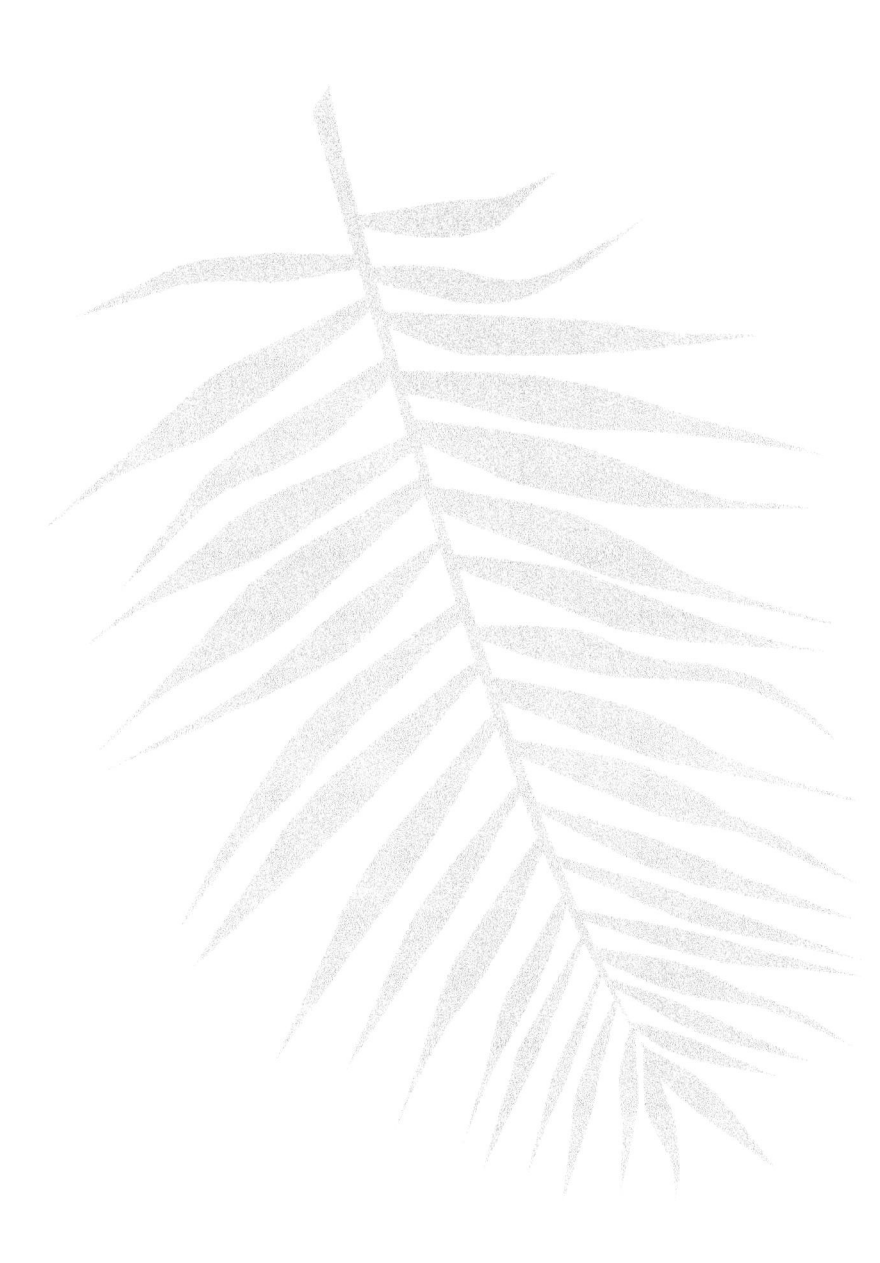

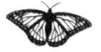
Chapter Sixteen

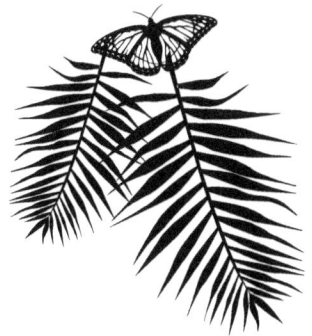

People wait and silently pray for someone to speak. Others speak but are not heard.

His name was Johamad.

The small village in which he lived was located in an isolated region in northern Madagascar. He was a soft spoken, gentle man well into his eighties and served as the village healer. Although he was a father, grandfather, and great-grandfather, Johamad was most commonly known by everyone in the village as *"Dada,"* which translated as 'Daddy.'

From the first moment we met, I knew he was special.

Of the inhabitants on Planet Earth, medicine men like Johamad are considered to be an endangered group. The indigenous knowledge and wisdom that a healer like Johamad possesses has been passed from father to son for as long as any can recall. Sadly, the information that has been transferred for generations is becoming lost to history as younger generations are gravitating toward more "Western" ways of life and away from tribal customs and traditions.

When anyone in their village needed treatment for a medical condition, they went to Johamad. As an experienced elder and healer, he could treat anything from constipation to a cough and from infections to asthma.

To our team, Johamad was also quite the ladies' man. Even though he was well into his eighth decade of life, he described his several wives and many children, grandchildren and great-grandchildren before bragging about his new wife, whom he described as a lovely young girl in her twenties. Sighing, he then complained that he needed to gather more medicine to give him the energy to keep up with her.

For five days, we hiked with Johamad, exploring the lands surrounding his village. He walked with bare feet and with hands behind his back, lightly clutching his handmade machete, while leading us over dry, arid lands and around lush marshes. Every so often, he stopped to describe a plant, tree or flower that he used for medicine.

During a hike one day, Johamad pointed to a thick bush. Seven feet tall and four feet wide, the shrub had copious swirling wooden stems, which were sparsely covered in slender, two-inch green leaves. Through a translator, he explained that within the soft, flexible vine-like stems were medicine, but not all parts of the plant were "good medicine." Some portions were immature and inactive and, therefore, ineffective.

Reaching out as far as he could toward the top of the shrub, Johamad gently cut off a section of the supple wooden stems with his machete. Holding it out for us to see, he described that he used the sap to treat eye irritations and infections.

When he said "eye," I cringed.

Chapter Sixteen

In the United States, pharmacists and medical professionals are very careful about medications for the eye, ensuring that they are sterile and free from contamination. Johamad, on the other hand, went into detail about placing the untreated liquid contents of the plant, which was growing in a deciduous forest, directly in the eye.

With the freshly cut ten-inch segment in his hand, he began squeezing it from one end to the other. Maintaining pressure, he continued to squeeze until his fingers reached the opposite end. Slowly, a small amount of liquid began to ooze out. It was as if he was squeezing a straw to get a few drops of liquid from one end to the other.

Collecting the drips of clear sap onto his index finger, he tilted his head back and placed his finger with the medicine in the corner of his right eye. It was a simple treatment, and he claimed that after a few days of use it would rid any infection and calm any irritation.

As I thought about the treatment, which had been used for generations, I wondered how the first healer had learned of it. Did he try it on a cut or scrape and then decide to try it in the eye? Had there been a vision or a dream or some form of spiritual guidance that led him to use the plant? Johamad did not know.

Johamad's knowledge of local plants was expansive and it seemed that he had a treatment for everything.

Except for weight loss.

When I asked if he had a treatment for losing weight, he remained silent for a moment with a perplexed look on his face before responding to the translator. The translator then asked me if it was to lose weight or to help someone gain weight. When I reiterated that it was to lose weight, Johamad shook his head no and explained that there is never a need for someone to lose weight, only to gain weight. Puzzled, he stated again that he could not understand why anyone would need medicine to lose weight.

During the second day in Johamad's village, late in the evening, my friend and our sound director, Alec, came to my hut about a problem. On every trip, there had been at least two or three team members who became sick for a short period of time or had a medical issue. Alec seemed to be the one to confront some of the most difficult issues.

Before every trek, I insisted that anytime anyone began to feel bad—headache, fever, aches, constipation, diarrhea, etcetera—that they let me know immediately. Things could take a quick turn for the worse; therefore, it was imperative that we be proactive and take care of things as soon as possible.

In my hut, Alec turned his back to me, slowly pulled down his pants and pointed to the backs of his legs. Intense redness and inflammation covered a six-inch-wide area which extended from his hamstrings across the back of his knees to the top of his gastrocnemii. It was like a horrific case of poison ivy or poison sumac, but worse. Because Alec had initially thought the skin reaction was a minor issue, he had not deemed it significant. But it had quickly worsened.

Bending down to take a closer look, my worry escalated as I saw hundreds of tiny blisters within the raised areas of his flesh. Although his skin was primarily bright red, there were several small regions, reddish-brown in color, that looked like second degree burns.

It was impossible to know the cause of the reaction because during the hikes we had frequently walked through thick brush and growth, trekking through sections that forced us to brush up against a variety of plants and trees. Even though most of us wore

Chapter Sixteen

shorts, we received only minor scrapes and cuts, and, unlike Alec, fared much better.

There were two choices. We could immediately start the prednisone tablets and triamcinolone cream, which were in our medical kits, or we could wait and ask Johamad for help in the morning. The prednisone tablets and the triamcinolone cream were both corticosteroids and would help calm the allergic response, the inflammation and itching.

But without hesitation, Alec insisted on asking Johamad, believing that he would know the local plants and best how to treat the reaction.

The following morning, Johamad was immediately shown the back of Alec's legs. Looking closely with furrowed brow, he announced that we must go for a walk to gather the medicine he needed.

We followed Johamad for well over two hours before he stopped walking and began to discuss the small group of plants he stood beside. The plants that would be the medicine for Alec's legs. With opposite leaves along their two-foot-tall stems, the plants were sturdy and so tough that it was impossible to pull them up by their roots or break them apart with human hands. As I used a Swiss Army knife, Johamad used his machete to cut multiple stems near the ground until we collected several handfuls.

As he collected the plants, Johamad explained that Alec's skin problem was a reaction to rubbing up against a poisonous plant. It was an issue that he had treated many times.

Later, when I researched allergic skin reactions, I learned that the chemical that likely caused Alec's reaction is found in the mango fruit's skin as well as in the cashew nut, both of which grow in Madagascar. The chemical, known as urushiol, is also the culprit for the allergic reactions that people have from poison ivy, poison oak and poison sumac.

Almost two hours later, we returned to Johamad's hut where he began preparing the treatment for Alec. Pulling the leaves off the stems, he placed them in the bottom of the largest mortar and pestle I had ever seen. The mortar was twelve inches in diameter and fifteen inches high, while the pestle was more like a large club, four feet in length.

Holding the pestle erect and close to his shoulder, Johamad pounded the plants until they were ground into a dark greenish-brown mush that looked like gobs of wet spinach. He then scraped the sides and the bottom of the mortar and placed the clump of moist leaves in the middle of a small swatch of thin cloth. Folding the edges of the fabric together, he picked it up and held it inches above Alec's affected areas, slowly squeezing the bundle until drops of juice trickled out.

Johamad then gently spread the liquid over the backs of Alec's legs, coloring his white skin yellowish-brown.

For the next several days, Johamad used various plants to create three separate treatments, corresponding to the different symptoms that Alec experienced. The first recipe Johamad used (the plant giving the yellowish-brown liquid) helped to calm the inflammation and diminish the itching. The second one, which was created by combining three different plants, helped to dry and heal the skin. And the third and final recipe, composed of yet another mixture of plants, including turmeric, helped to completely heal the skin and prevent scarring.

In all my years as a pharmacist, I had recommended treatments for poison oak and ivy hundreds of times, yet I had never considered using such an elaborate regimen with multiple treatments to

Chapter Sixteen

tackle the different stages and symptoms. In the U.S., there are a variety of products. Some are to dry the skin, some to also target itching and even others to prevent the urushiol from binding to the skin. But typically, one product is selected and used until the condition improves.

Johamad's approach to Alec's problem was brilliant. He not only focused on easing Alec's discomfort but also on healing the skin. And this urushiol remedy was only one of many treatments that he shared; he also showed us treatments that included medicine for worms, wounds, pain and tremors. His medical knowledge was so deep and vast that we barely scratched the surface of what he knew.

And we weren't the only ones who failed to grasp the breadth of his knowledge.

Surprisingly, there was not one person in the village who cared to learn from him and continue the traditions of their forefathers. His sons had chosen to pursue more western ways of life, while others in the village had no desire to follow in Johamad's footsteps as a healer. With no written records and with a discontinuation of the oral traditions, Johamad's knowledge and wisdom would most likely disappear when he did.

The villagers could not understand our focus and attention on Johamad. Even Johamad had initially been surprised by it. However, he claimed it brought him great joy that we wanted to listen and learn from him. He took pride in helping his village, and it made him very happy that he might also help others, even if they were from lands far away.

Over those few days, I became very close to Johamad. We talked about his family and the changes he had seen in his life, changes that included family members moving away from the village and the destruction of nearby lands for wood and for rice fields. He spoke of the young boys and girls in the village who longed to live in the capital city of Antananarivo, where there were jobs and money and things to buy. We spoke of life in the United States as I shared stories of my family and friends and described things like movies, french fries and snow.

When it was time for us to leave, it was difficult to say good-bye. Our team had bonded with the village and, for me, saying good-bye to Johamad was like saying good-bye to a dear friend.

Before our arrival, it seemed that little attention had been given to Johamad in his role as their healer. But with our focus on him, it appeared that the village began to sense his importance. Regardless of what happened when we departed, I believe Johamad realized that a part of him would be carried with us, across many thousands of miles, never to be forgotten.

Return treks to a country were dictated by funding and were typically instigated by the for-profit company, Natural Discoveries, with plant collections for research. Although the return treks focused on research, the non-profit always seized the opportunity to send along at least one person to film, in order to capture additional footage for educational materials.

For Madagascar, the first follow-up trip was almost three years later. Because money was tight with the for-profit, we could only afford to send one person, who would then join with our guide in Madagascar to travel to see the healers. As my business partner returned that year to further our work in the field, I remained at the pharmacy to earn money to fund the company.

Chapter Sixteen

Three years later, after my partner's trip, I finally had the opportunity to return to Madagascar. It had been six years since I was there, and I was most excited to see Johamad. I had carefully prepared gifts for him such as flashlights, matches, an expedition shirt, dry bags and chocolates, as well as photos that we had taken during the trip six years earlier.

The guide who had helped us with the two previous treks had taken a job with a Madagascar company and could not take the three weeks off to travel. I, however, found another guide, Angelo, with the help of the Madagascar Consulate. Angelo was in his early thirties. He was polite and courteous, and his English was good. With his help, I bought plane tickets to fly north, hired a driver, rented a Land Cruiser, and we made our way to the region where Johamad lived.

After traveling for two days, we neared the vicinity of Johamad's village. The area had changed dramatically and was vastly different from what I recalled. The once sparsely populated area with its long, quiet stretch of road had been transformed into a bustling community with abundant huts, roadside stands and a dense population.

I searched for the only landmark I knew . . . Johamad's sheltered hut. With a thatched v-shaped roof and no walls, the simple seven-by-seven-foot covered structure was the place where we sat every day for hours talking with Johamad.

As the vehicle inched along the road, I looked intently toward the land on the left side until I finally spotted the shelter. Slightly hidden by the overgrowth of seedlings and plant life, the structure sat catty-corner to a hut and twenty-five yards from the road. Sections of its thatched roof were missing, exposing the few remaining rotten floor boards to the elements. It appeared long-abandoned and long-forgotten.

The driver pulled off the side of the road, and, with Angelo and me, walked over to two young women selling bananas and papayas at a nearby stand. Asking if they would direct us to Johamad, the women turned to each other, spoke in Malagasy and then shrugged, claiming they knew no one by the name. The driver then walked a few steps further and asked three other women the same question but got the same response. He then turned to ask a man who stood only a few feet beyond them, yet the man also shook his head no.

No one knew a man named Johamad.

Thinking perhaps it was my pronunciation, I gave variations of the name, asking if there was a Johamatra or Johamata. But again, we received the same disappointing response. I continued by describing him, explaining that he was the healer . . . the medicine man. As I talked and Angelo translated, I pulled out the photos I had brought as a gift for Johamad and passed them around. But still, no one recognized him. No one knew him.

Others started to gather as Angelo and several women continued to ask and pass around the photos. Sadly, not one person could offer any assistance.

I couldn't believe what I was hearing. It had only been six years. And actually, it had only been a little over three since my business partner had visited the place and spent time with Johamad. How could it be that a healer who treated so many and who had many wives and children had suddenly disappeared?

As the crowd became larger, the driver, Angelo and I continued to inquire. It seemed everyone wanted to help, but no one could. Finally, a young man stepped forward and said that he knew Johamad. Johamad was his grandfather.

He was a young man in his early twenties, strong and physically fit with beautiful, thick black hair. He was shy and yet confident, and his name was Hasina.

Chapter Sixteen

I held out the photos, and as Hasina stared at them, he nodded his head yes. Smiling, I extended my hand and we shook hands. Angelo explained that I was a friend of his grandfather who had traveled from the United States of America to visit Johamad. Angelo elaborated that many years ago, my team had spent many days with his grandfather to learn about his culture and his plant medicines.

Hasina smiled. And asked us to follow him.

As we followed him along a narrow dirt path, I asked Angelo to translate how excited I was to return and spend time with Johamad . . . that he had always been very special to me . . . that Johamad was one of my most favorites. While I continued to talk, the grandson spoke very little and only turned around slightly to nod, acknowledging Angelo's words.

The short five-minute walk led us to a small hut. I was overwhelmed with emotion, eager to see Johamad again. Excited to hug him and thrilled to spend more time with him.

Inside the hut, Hasina introduced us to his wife, explaining to her who we were and that we had come to see Johamad. With an almost blank expression, she nodded slightly and smiled. Hasina then looked down at the ground before slowly raising his head to say that he was sad to tell us that his grandfather had died one year earlier.

I stood motionless and struggled to fight back the tears.

Hasina then went over to the corner of the room to a stack of clothes and odd items. Placing the clothes and other items off to the side, he unveiled a book which had been buried underneath. He carefully picked up the book and began to describe it as a family heirloom, stating that the book had important papers, writings, pieces of cloth and other treasured items.

And the Silent Spoke

Walking back to where we were standing, he opened the bulging eleven-by-fourteen-inch book and thumbed through its pages. He then tapped on one of the pages and asked if the photo of the man was the one we were seeking. Turning the book around so that Angelo and I could see, he pointed to a photo in the top left-hand corner.

No longer able to hold back the tears, I looked up at him and nodded yes. The photo, he said, was one of only a few pictures their family had, and it was one of only three photos of Johamad.

The picture brought back waves of memories. He wore the same multi-colored shirt of green, burgundy, white and yellow and posed with the same walking stick he had used every day we had walked with him. Freckles dotted his cheeks, while the same beard with its shadow of white whiskers stood prominent against his smooth brown skin.

Mostly though, I remembered his eyes, caring and gentle, which seemed to glisten when he smiled. Everything about the photo brought back memories. He was exactly as I remembered.

For in the photo, standing next to him . . .

Was me.

When Hasina realized that I was the one in the photo with Johamad, he kept repeating, "It is you. It is you with my grandfather." And then he made a comment that my hair had turned much whiter since the photo was taken. And laughed.

He flipped the page to look at the other two photos of Johamad and then laughed with excitement. Turning the book around for us to see, he pointed at the two photos and then at me. The photos were of Johamad standing with our entire team.

It had been during my business partner's return trip a few years earlier that the three photos had been given to Johamad as a gift.

Chapter Sixteen

Turning to his wife, Hasina asked that she gather the children and family.

As each family member arrived, Hasina pointed to the photos and proudly announced that I was a friend of his grandfather's. When the children gathered, he took the book and, squatting amongst them, pointed to the photos and described the man as his grandfather. And me, as his grandfather's friend. When everyone had arrived, Hasina continued by telling the children and adults that I had traveled many miles and across the sea to see his grandfather again.

And with pride, Hasina said that his grandfather had been a very important man.

With Angelo translating, I spoke about the days that our team had spent with Johamad and how much I honored and cherished his friendship. Although I tried not to cry, tears filled my eyes.

I then gave Hasina the gifts I had brought for Johamad, including several other photos from the trip six years earlier. They were pictures gathering plants, sitting under the shelter and one of Johamad as he turned to walk the road back home on the day we said good-bye.

After passing the photos around for everyone to see, Hasina placed them next to the others in the folds of the book.

And carefully closed it.

Before leaving, Angelo took several group photos of me with Johamad's offspring, including with Hasina and his immediate family, other grandchildren and great-grandchildren. As we stood together with arms around one another, I glanced around at the individuals in the group.

I saw Johamad in their smiles and in their eyes. I saw his gentleness and his compassion. And I could only imagine how proud he would have been to be standing there as well.

Back in the SUV, I barely uttered a word for hours. The sadness was indescribable, and as the emotions became stronger, the tears began to flow. The tears were for the friend I would never see again and for the village who never knew his name. And they were for the world who would fail to learn the gifts he had never been asked to share.

I picked up my camera and looked through the photos that only hours earlier had been taken. A multitude of memories and thoughts began to swarm, but one thought lingered foremost in my heart and mind. Johamad's death was not only the death of a wonderful man and a deeply gifted healer, it was the death and demise of hundreds and possibly thousands of years of wisdom and knowledge.

And unbeknownst to him or to his community, and to most of the world, he had been a most priceless and endangered member of the human race.

Chapter Seventeen

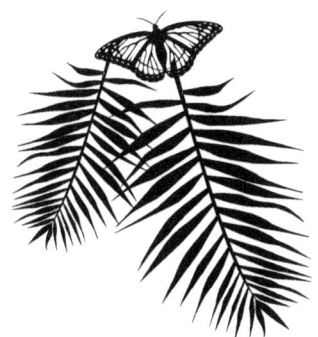

Many forms of life on Planet Earth continue to disappear at an alarming rate. Cultures, species and land. The escalating loss has created an ever-growing global campaign to encourage better protection, more sustainable practices and conscious development. In Madagascar, many regions of land are being destroyed not only by such outside forces as logging and mining, but also by the practices of the Malagasy people.

The loss has taken a tremendous toll.

According to NASA, as much as ninety percent of Madagascar's original forests has been destroyed in the last century.

From planes, we looked down upon barren lands that had once been thriving forests. In our SUVs, we peered out over land that was so dry it looked like desert. The ground was at times beige, at times red and other times black from being charred by fires. Not only had the lush vegetation been destroyed, but countless biological species.

As I bore witness to this devastation, I couldn't help but wonder if it was possible for the land to ever return to its former natural state. And if so, how many generations would pass before it could be restored?

One of the primary reasons for the man-made destruction in Madagascar is an agricultural practice called 'slash and burn,' which the locals called *"tavy."* In the practice of tavy, an area of forest is cut and burned in order to use the land for agriculture. As a result, blackened carcasses of land dot the countryside, appearing void of life except for a handful of small charred trees.

According to our Malagasy guide, Yupi, when the land is cleared, it is often used to create rice paddies. After a couple years of rice, the land is left idle for five or six years. After this idle period, the land is used again to grow rice for a couple of years before once again being left fallow. At the end of the second or third rotation, the nutrients in the soil have become so depleted that the land can support but little life.

Land is also cleared for grass to grow in order to feed the zebu. According to Yupi, the Malagasy people consider the forests unlimited. When a piece of land is exhausted, they simply move to another area of forest and repeat the process.

In the southwestern part of the country, Yupi explained, the Malagasy people destroy the land by chopping down trees to use the wood primarily to make charcoal. Without other means of energy such as electricity, charcoal is the main energy source and many people make their livelihoods from making and selling it.

Family members sit for hours alongside roads or at the market

Chapter Seventeen

with piles of coal stacked in the shape of pyramids, hoping to sell a few pieces. Sometimes the sales mean the difference between eating or not.

Some of the best trees they use for charcoal are located in the Spiny Forest, a unique ecosystem found nowhere else in the world. As the demand for charcoal has grown, the trees of the Spiny Forest have been utilized, and as a result, areas of the vibrant forest have slowly disappeared.

Both practices (slash and burn and charcoal production) leave the lands barren and nutrient-poor. The soil is no longer anchored by the roots of trees and other vegetation, and therefore, is easily washed away with the heavy rains.

And the process of erosion begins.

Erosion in Madagascar has reached such a critical level that the run-off has turned the rivers, streams and sections of the Indian Ocean bright red. Astronauts claim that from space Madagascar looks like it is bleeding to death. The run-off into the ocean causes sediment to coat fish eggs and destroy many other life forms. Including those within the coral reefs.

After passing several areas of destroyed lands during a full day of travel in our SUV, we arrived at the place where we would overnight. The land where we pitched our tents was owned by the father of one of Yupi's friends.

As we made camp, I recalled the sights we had seen throughout the day's travel. The practices of unsustainably using natural resources are not only Malagasy issues; they are global issues. The devastation we witnessed was as alarming as the environmental

And the Silent Spoke

issues that are confronted in other parts of the world, from uncontrolled logging and mining practices, overdevelopment and mountain top removal to the daunting stress of an ever-increasing and unsustainable human population.

Conversations with team members that night dwelled on these issues and the feelings each of us had about the demise of the land. Madagascar was such a beautiful country, yet the giant swaths of land that were being destroyed were heart-wrenching. We spoke of other treasures in the world that were also under threat—places like the Great Barrier Reef and the Amazon as well as our own communities, where thousands of acres of land had been and were continuing to be cleared for development. Rivers polluted by chemicals, air tainted with emissions, and lands and waters littered with non-biodegradable materials like plastics.

Fertile lands that were once utilized for fishing, hunting, gathering and a myriad of other things continue to disappear . . . and with the loss, plants and medicines used for hundreds and possibly thousands of years.

We talked at length before slowly shifting focus to marvel at the evening sky.

It was a spectacularly clear evening and the constellations were surreal. Millions of flickering stars for as far as the eye could see. I reveled in the sky's expansiveness and yet, was greatly humbled by my microscopic presence.

As with most evenings on expedition, I was the first person to turn in for the night. Maybe it was my age, as I had a good twelve years on the others, or maybe it was simply that I seized the opportunity to sleep when it was possible. Regardless, I crawled inside my small two-man tent and zipped it up. The temperature had dropped slightly over the past couple of hours, so I put on a

Chapter Seventeen

mid-weight base layer shirt and pants before stretching across the thin sleeping pad and quickly falling asleep.

Only to soon awaken. And awaken cold.

Thinking that the thin silk bivy sack would be appropriate and comfortable for this leg of the trek, I had opted not to bring a sleeping bag. The southern region had daytime temperatures close to ninety degrees Fahrenheit. Because of the high temperatures, I chose to leave my warmer clothing and sleeping bag behind at the last drop point with other equipment and supplies.

What I didn't realize about this area was that the temperature dropped dramatically at night, often into the fifties. What I had packed was inadequate to handle the evening temperature plunges.

Grabbing my headlamp, I rummaged through my backpack and pulled out all of my clothes. I quickly put on three of the four shirts I had packed and a pair of wool socks. I took the fourth shirt and wrapped it snuggly around my head, covering my ears and most of my face, and then curled into the fetal position.

The layers brought a little warmth, but I was still cold. It was ten o'clock at night and was going to get much colder as the night went on. I couldn't help but to feel sorry for myself, wishing that I had brought the sleeping bag. Longing for warmer clothes.

The pity I had for myself quickly changed as I thought of the team and our guides. Were they warm? Were they okay? They had packed as I had and surely would experience the same coldness.

I thought of the Malagasy people and the children. The majority we had encountered had limited clothing and most had never owned a pair of shoes. How did they stay warm? What was it like to be a parent watching their children shiver night after night?

Suddenly I understood one of the reasons why the Malagasy people were utilizing their land in the way that they were. Timber was vital for the fires that kept their families warm and provided the heat for cooking and preparing food, thus helping to ensure their survival. Their short-term needs were basic needs, and they took great precedence over any possible long-term consequences of the environment, preservation and sustainability. Such futuristic matters about saving the environment were irrelevant and inconceivable.

Earlier in the trek, my thoughts and opinions about the expansive deforestation had been focused on protecting the environment. But I soon found myself embarrassed and ashamed that I had judged the Malagasy people for taking the very actions that were helping them to survive. Why would they be concerned about the environment—about the next week, the next year, the future and future generations—when they were only trying to make it day to day?

The evenings of shivering in my tent would forever change the way I looked at the practices and actions of others. My thoughts had been based on the world that I knew, with limited insight and perspective of the world at large.

With a life of safeties, amenities, comforts and even luxuries, I could never truly fathom the world of those whom I witnessed from a distance. Their situations and circumstances varied to such extents that to even have an opinion about their actions without deeper awareness and acumen was both short-sighted and insensitive.

It was easy for me to look at others and at circumstances with an outside perspective, to form judgments and conclusions. The challenge was to stop the thoughts within my own mind and to instead listen and try to first understand the perspectives of others and their journeys.

Chapter Seventeen

If you are lucky, there will be opportunities to walk side by side with some very special people, if only for a moment in time. If you are blessed, you will gain deeper insight into their lives, their pilgrimages . . . and their truths.

At that point, a part of them becomes imbedded into your soul . . .

And you are never the same.

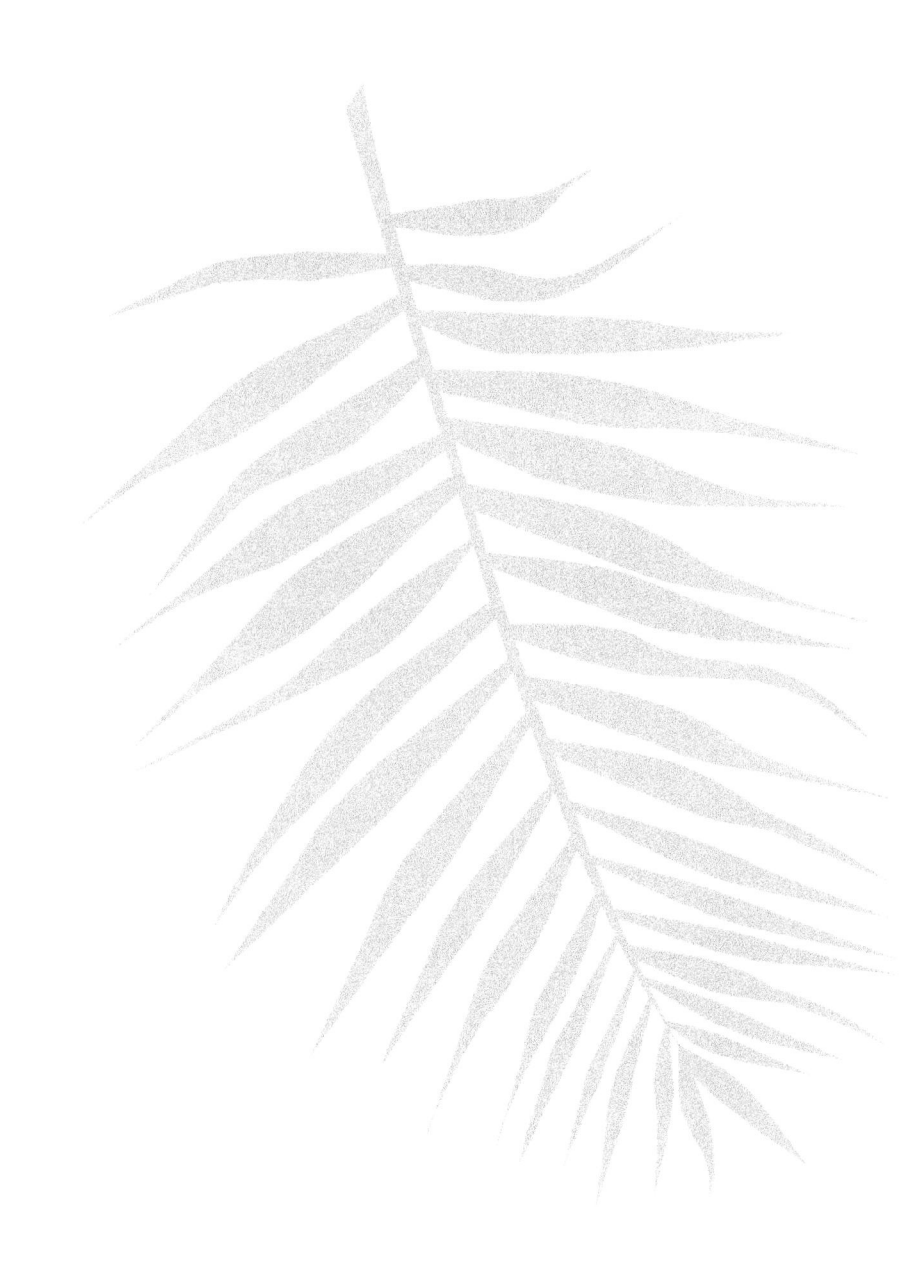

Chapter Eighteen

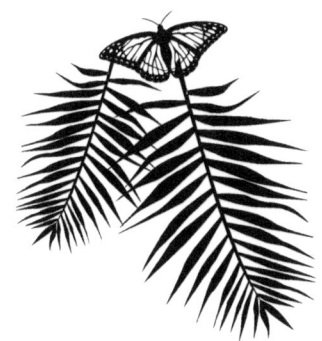

It was nearing her bedtime, and although she tried to stay awake, she was too tired. As much as she enjoyed being with her nieces and nephews, the talking exhausted her. Closing her eyes, she relaxed in their company as she had the evening before.

The smell of barbecue permeated the room. Sandwiches made of the famous North Carolina pork had always been one of the kids' favorites, and she took great delight in seeing their excitement when Dominga entered the room carrying a tray piled high.

She, on the other hand, had not had much of an appetite for days. And it didn't matter.

After the sandwiches, hushpuppies and slaw, the nieces and nephews raved about the lemon pound cake and Swiss chocolate torte. The Swiss chocolate torte, another of her mother's special recipes, was her personal favorite since childhood.

While the kids ate, she spoke only a few more words.

I'm sorry if I have rambled too much today. I hope that I haven't bored you. Your time with me has brought great joy to my heart, a joy that has been missing for far too long.

I realize that you will all be going back home tomorrow. It will be sad for me. So, in case I am too emotional tomorrow to say so, I want to tell you how much I love you, how proud I am of you and how honored I am to be your aunt.

I wish for you lives overflowing with serenity and love. I wish for you wisdom to follow your own paths and to walk your truths. May you explore the world beyond, but more importantly, the world within. And in the process, discover those things which feed your soul.

Please understand that you are never alone. Even if you are not aware of it, you are guided and protected by many who will always love you. Both here and in the beyond.

There is still a little more I would like to share with you in the morning, if you would be so kind. But for now, I am tired and need to rest, as the energy that once ran through this body is no longer to be found.

One by one, her nieces and nephews gently kissed her and said goodnight. While she retired to her bedroom, the kids remained in the room as they had done the evening before—eating, drinking and talking. Although her bedroom was at the opposite end of the house, she continued to hear their every word, almost as if they were only a few feet away.

She was exhausted yet could not sleep.

Over the past few months, there had been more and more sleepless nights. Her body appeared to relax, remaining completely still, but her mind refused to quieten. Listening to the tick-tock of the clock by her bedside, she

Chapter Eighteen

would lie on her side and stare at the unrelenting movement of the clock's hands, thinking about her life . . . until she would finally drift into sleep.

Since the nieces and nephews had arrived, however, she had become even more restless. After finally falling asleep, noises would abruptly awaken her, even in the early morning hours when everyone should be sleeping.

Sometimes, the noises were beeping sounds like that of an alarm or a truck backing up. At other times, they were like muffled voices. With a house full of guests and a plethora of technical devices, it was not surprising, especially since several of the nieces and nephews were in different time zones and had to attend to business.

Regardless, the sudden jolts into wakefulness startled and unraveled her, making it difficult to relax and nearly impossible to get a decent night's rest.

She was eighty-nine years old. It equated to almost forty-seven million minutes . . . approximately seven hundred and eighty thousand hours. Over thirty-two thousand days.

It was an enormous amount of time, the majority of which she could not recount. For her, time had been mysterious, and, like a magician, it seemed to have made the hours, days and years disappear right before her eyes.

Regardless, the journey had been good to her. It had only been in the past nine months that her health had dramatically declined, and her body had drastically weakened. She could no longer drive, and she required assistance with most things, including cooking and cleaning.

For seven days a week, Dominga had been there for her, becoming not only her caretaker, but her friend.

It had been Dominga who had meticulously cleaned and prepped for the kids' arrival, preparing all the food during the days prior. Without

Dominga, the pampering and the special things she had planned would not have been possible.

It was hard to believe the three days were coming to an end. It would be difficult to say good-bye. The thought alone of the kids leaving made her weep.

For she knew tomorrow would be unlike any other good-bye.

Tomorrow would likely be the final good-bye.

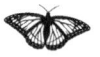

Chapter Nineteen

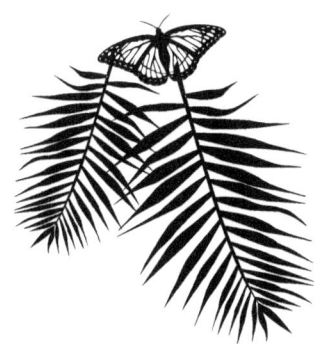

She awakened early, and to her surprise, so had her nieces and nephews. As the kids made their way to the kitchen, Dominga created their favorite lattes and coffees, given special attention to every detail. Whiffs of vanilla and cinnamon mingled with the aroma of freshly ground coffee, engulfing the room.

She was going to miss that. And them.

A lot.

With mugs in hand, they made their way to the living room and gathered around her as they had done the two days before. A few minutes later, Dominga passed around a plate of warm scones and, being the ever-diligent caretaker, quietly inquired about her morning medications. Because there were so many things that she depended on Dominga to do for her, she insisted that she alone would take care of her medications. She was, after all, a pharmacist for most of her life.

In the past several weeks, however, Dominga had noticed that the three bottles that were due for refills still had tablets remaining inside them. Of highest concern was her blood thinner, which helped to prevent blood clots and strokes.

Without giving any further thought to her medications, she turned her full attention to her nieces and nephews. And began another story.

It took three years to return to Papua New Guinea from the previous trek. Because of limited funds, instead of a six-member team, there was only a team of two. My dear friend and fellow explorer Eduardo, who had been with me since day one, would join me as we teamed up with our guide Jimson in Port Moresby to return to two of the areas we had originally explored. The first area would be the secluded island off the northern coast of Madang Province where Kupsey lived and the second, a remote jungle region near the western border of the Southern Highlands.

Two weeks before we departed the United States, I received an email from Jimson. In the email, he requested that we cancel the second leg of the trek because he felt the area was too dangerous. Instead, he recommended that we travel to his family village, which was in an isolated region in western Morobe Province.

In response, I typed that the guide company that we had hired years earlier had also advised avoiding the specific area of the Southern Highlands because they felt it was not safe. I imagined the area might be especially concerning to Jimson because he had never been to that part of the country. I assured him, however, that there was nothing to fear and that we had friends there, like Dexjo, whom we had hired during our first trip.

As I wrote, I wondered if Jimson was afraid of the small plane, which was piloted and operated by missionaries, or if he had an ulterior motive in changing the itinerary to his village so that his village would benefit financially from our visit. When we stayed

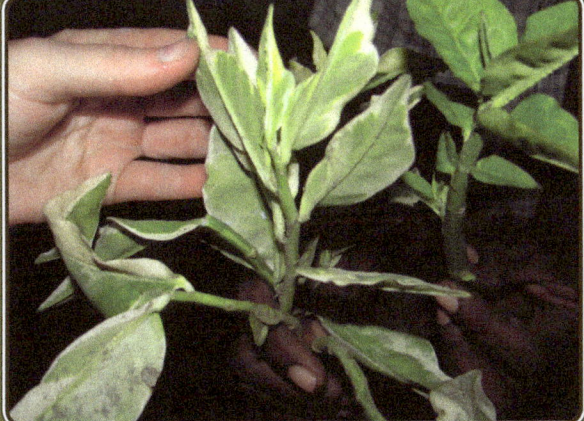

(Photo by Esteban Barrera)

Medicinal plants, Papua New Guinea

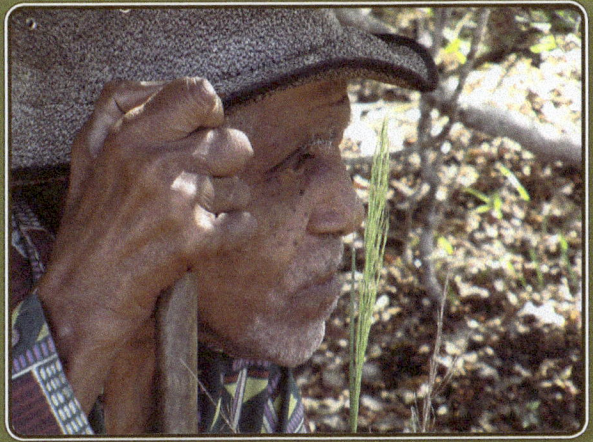

(Photo by Amy Greeson)

Malagasy Healer, Johamad

Chapter 16

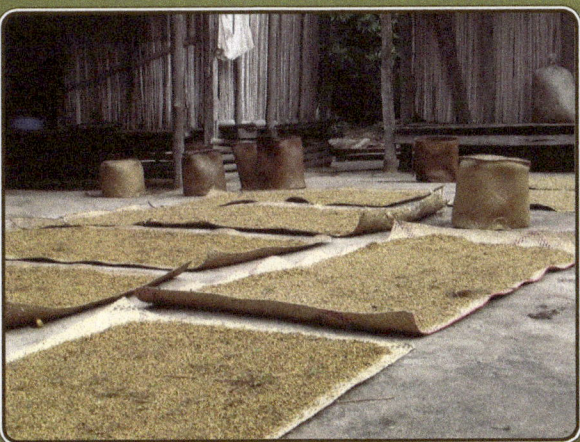

(Photo by Amy Greeson)

Village of Nirvana

Chapter 6

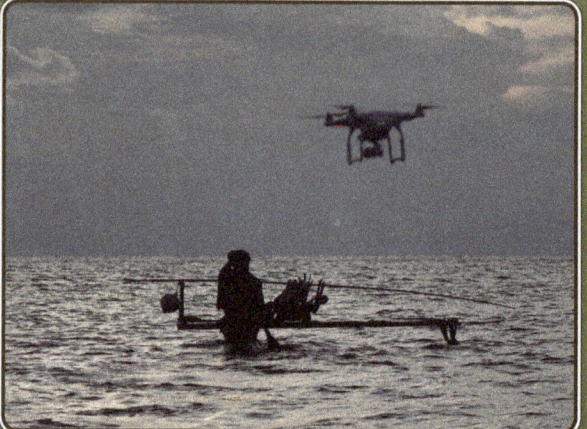

Fisherman and drone, near island off the coast of Papua New Guinea

Chapter 19

(Photo by Amy Greeson)

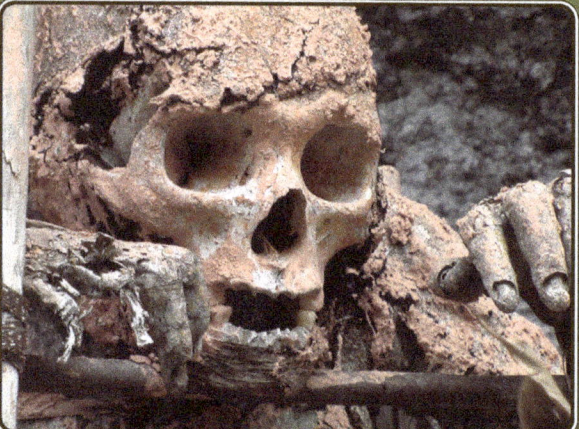

KukuKuku tribe, Papua New Guinea

Chapter 8

Goroka Show

Chapter 12

(Photo by Amy Greeson)

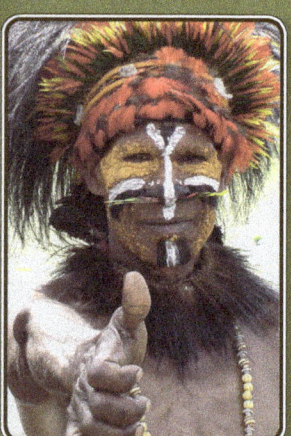 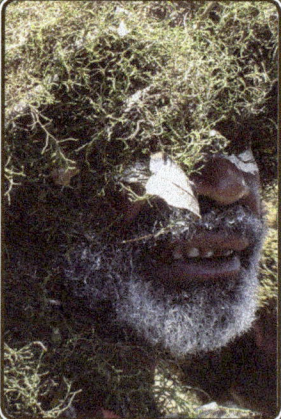

(Photos by Amy Greeson)

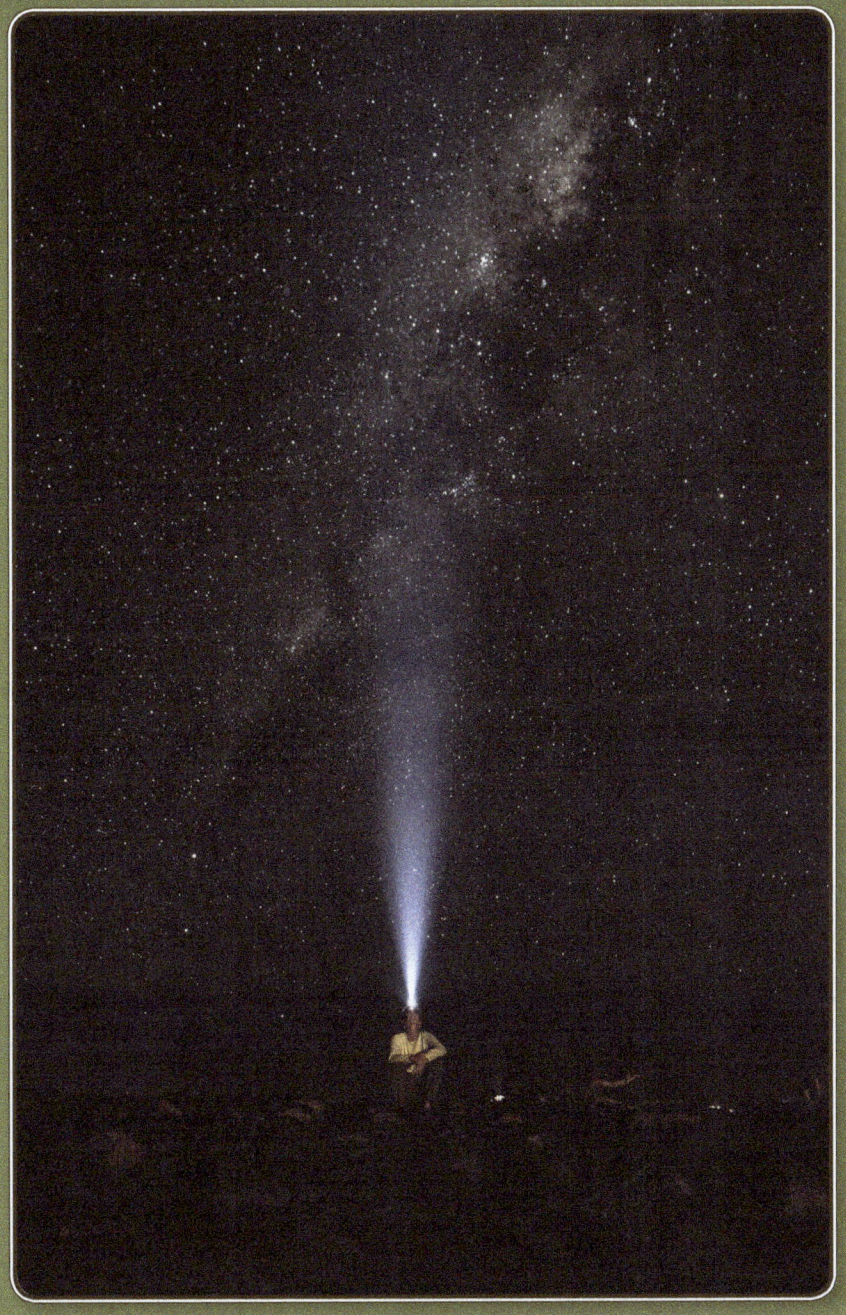

Amy under the Milky Way Galaxy, Madagascar

Chapter 17

(Photo by Esteban Barrera)

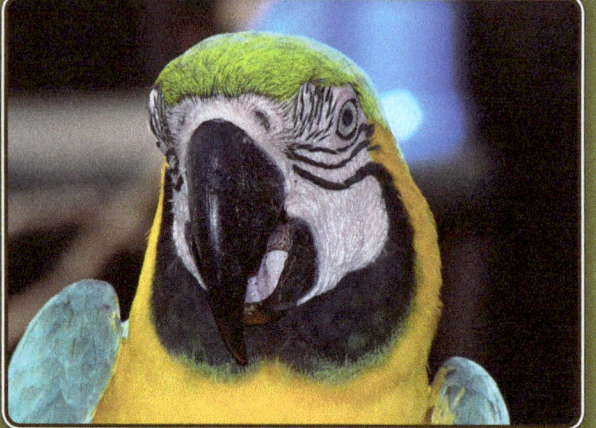

(Photo by Amy Greeson)

Blue & Gold
Macaw parrot, Amazon

Chapter 3

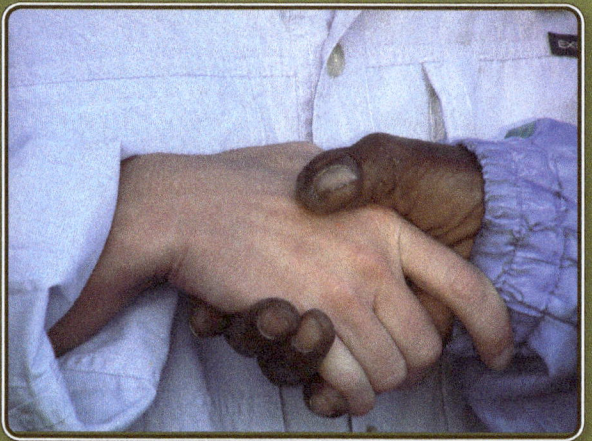

(Photo by Esteban Barrera)

Friendship, Madagascar

Chapter 20

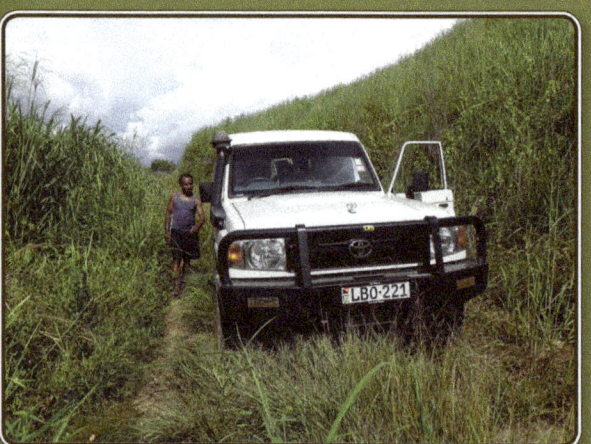

(Photo by Amy Greeson)

Searching for flying foxes
Papua New Guinea

Chapter 6

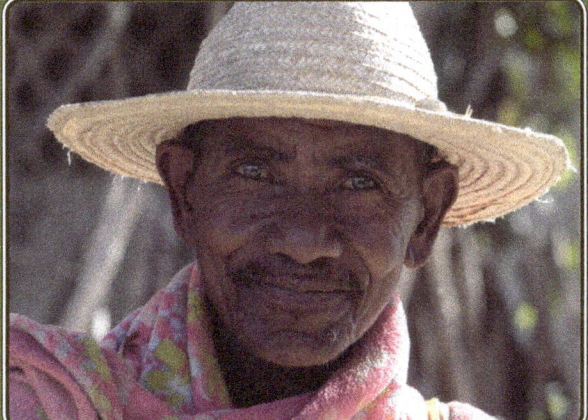

(Photo by Amy Greeson)

Madagascar

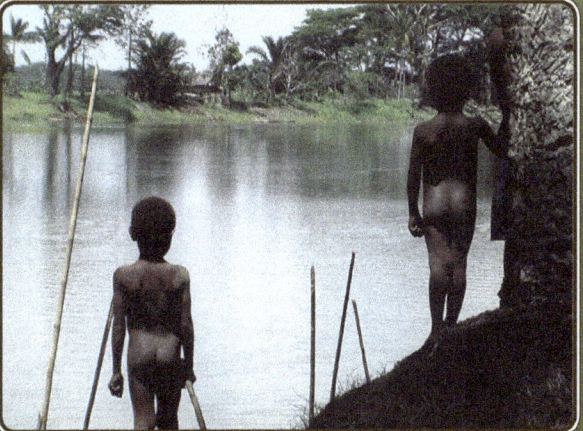

(Photo by Amy Greeson)

Sepik River,
Papua New Guinea

Chapter 15

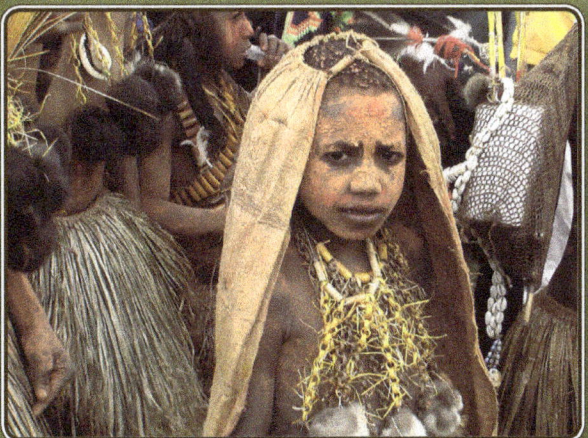

(Photo by Amy Greeson)

Goroka Show

Chapter 12

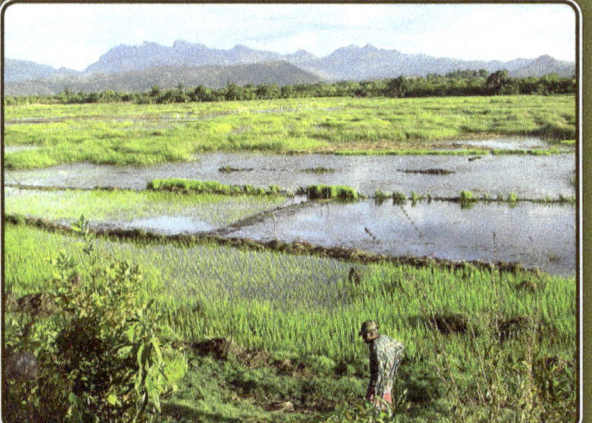

(Photo by Amy Greeson)

Rice fields, Madagascar

Chapter 17

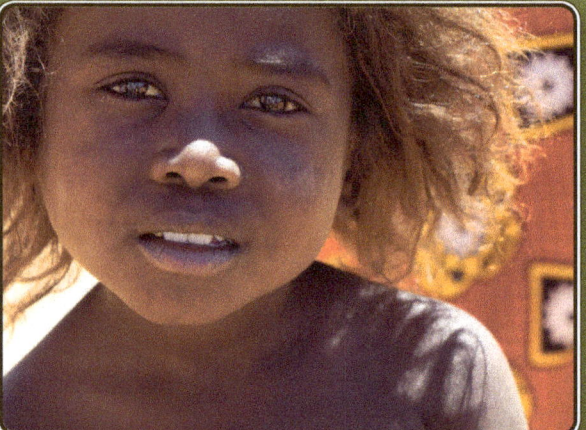

(Photo by Amy Greeson)

Madagascar

Chapter 17

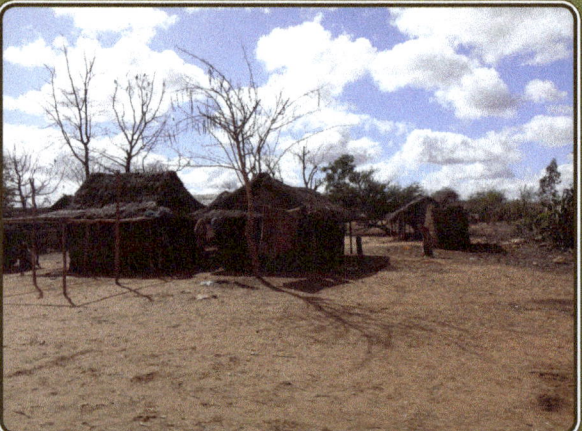

(Photo by Amy Greeson)

Madagascar

Chapter 17

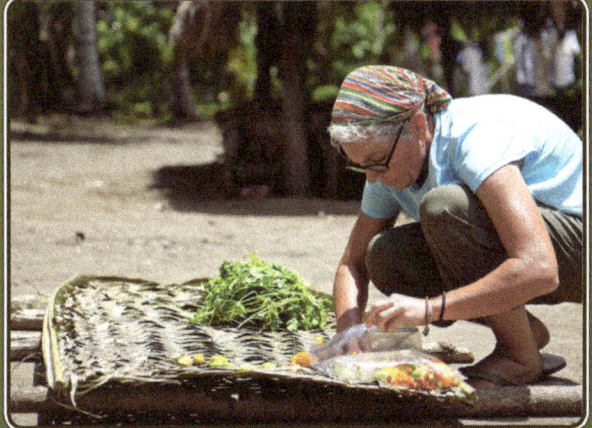

Spreading plants to dry, Papua New Guinea

(Photo by Esteban Barrera)

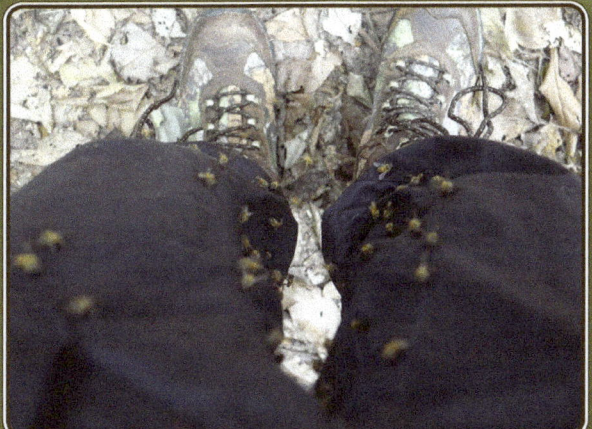

Swarms of bees, Republic of the Congo

Chapter 24

(Photo by Amy Greeson)

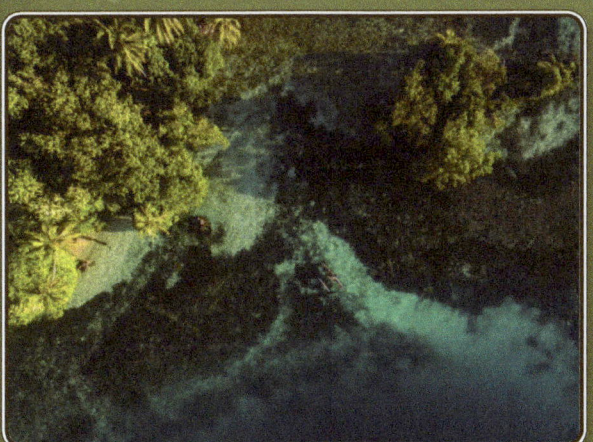

Island in the Bismarck Sea

Chapter 10

(Drone Photo by Esteban Barrera)

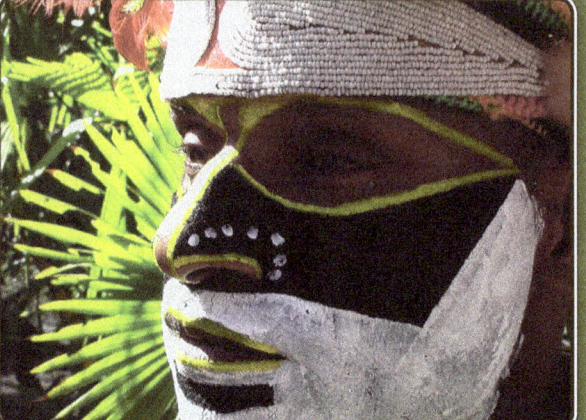

Goroka Show, Papua New Guinea

Chapter 21

(Photo by Amy Greeson)

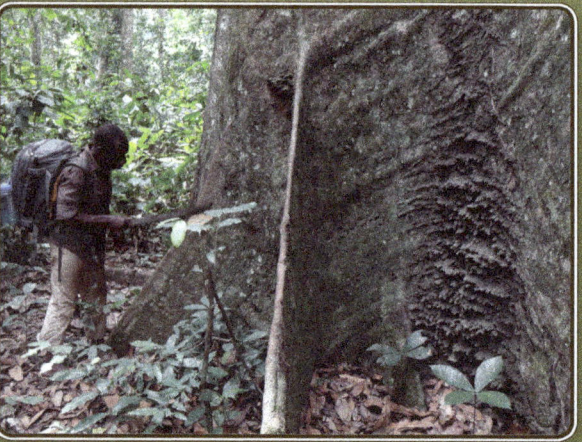

A tracker gathering bark for medicine, Republic of the Congo

Chapter 24

(Photo by Amy Greeson)

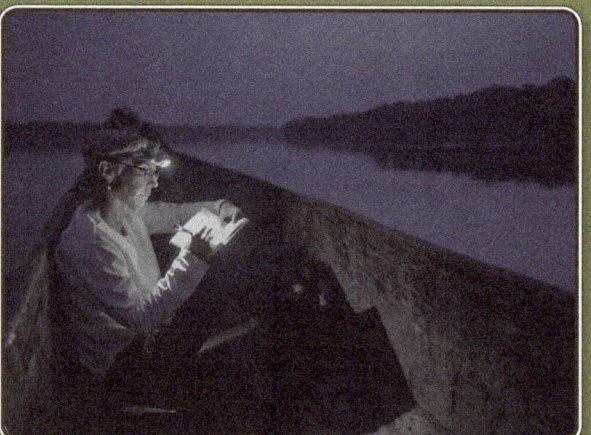

Traveling along the Sangha River before being arrested, Republic of the Congo

Chapter 27

(Photo by Esteban Barrera)

Chapter Nineteen

with a village, not only did we pay for lodging in a guesthouse or hut, we also paid for food, helpers and additional guides, as well as giving both money and other gifts such as machetes, dry bags and medical supplies, if needed, to the village.

Regardless, for several days Jimson and I went back and forth with numerous emails. As adamant as he was in his claims that the area was too dangerous and as persistent as he was with a change in plans, I was just as insistent that there was no reason to be afraid and that we should follow the set itinerary. Eventually, Jimson gave in . . . and agreed to do the trip as originally scheduled.

It took thirty-one hours for Eduardo and me to fly from the Raleigh-Durham airport in North Carolina to Port Moresby, Papua New Guinea. Jimson met us at the airport and, after dropping our bags at a small hotel, we walked to a nearby restaurant for dinner. We were less than fifteen minutes into our conversation when Jimson brought up the itinerary and the second region. He pleaded with us to cancel and instead allow him to take us to his family's village.

Frustrated by the thought of having to hash it out once again, I asked him to help me understand why he was so afraid. I knew that he thought the area was too dangerous, but he had never elaborated on why, and I had never specifically asked what scared him so much.

"There are many tribal disputes now," he said. "People are being killed. There is much hatred towards outsiders and white people. I am afraid that we might also be killed if we go there."

He paused.

"You see, some of the locals are upset about the natural gas project that is underway there. In the beginning, the project had been welcomed by the locals who eagerly agreed to sell their land to the oil and gas corporation and were excited about the money. However,

— 173 —

when the lands were bulldozed and cleared and when the money ran out, the people became angry. With their land partially barren and their 'home' destroyed, they had nothing to show for it."

Jimson then placed his hand gently on my forearm and said, "I know you will do what you want to do and what you feel you must do, but I hope that you will not go. It is not safe for any of us there . . . especially the two of you."

We continued to discuss the issue throughout dinner, debating the pros and cons and hearing more details from Jimson. The necessity to return to this particular region was based on one plant we had collected that had demonstrated a possible activity against cancer, in very early testing. How could we not go? How could we not try to help the millions of people who were desperate for such a cure? What if the plant only grew in this one region of the world? And what if the bulldozing and destruction with the current development was eradicating the species, and others? Only to be lost forever?

No matter how much I desired to collect the specimen, I could not put the lives of Eduardo and Jimson at such risk. Plus, if anything happened to us, there would not be any plants to bring back anyway.

Although I knew it was the right decision to follow Jimson's advice, I was hugely disappointed. In the best-case scenario, it would be another year before we could return because of the collection window. Plants needed to be collected at the same time each year to have the greatest chance of consistency. A change in season, temperature, rain, insects and other life forms mating or pollinating could theoretically alter a plant's constituents and compounds, and thus, its medicinal activity and potency.

After dinner and back at the hotel, I flopped across the bed. I was tired yet couldn't sleep. I continued thinking of the people

Chapter Nineteen

back home battling cancer and other horrific diseases. I thought of the many individuals I saw on a regular basis and others who were represented by the statistics cited in articles and journals. Statistics about life expectancy with current treatments and statistics about offspring battling the same conditions. By not collecting the specimen, I felt like I was failing them, their families and those who would face such battles in the years to come.

I also wondered if there was another reason we were being redirected for the second leg of the trek. Jimson spoke of powerful plant medicines that his family's village used and wanted to share with us. What if there were plants in this new region that needed our attention more?

Trusting that there was a reason and a purpose for why things were happening and believing that a higher power was directing us away from danger made it easier for me to accept the change.

The next day we embarked on the first part of the trek and headed north. Travel began with a one-hour flight to Lae, the capital of Morobe Province, which is also the second-largest city in Papua New Guinea. We arrived in time to buy a generator and fuel, necessary to recharge batteries and download footage. The three of us then went to the local grocery store and purchased supplies such as water, fruit, ramen noodles, rice and vegetables before finding a small hotel to overnight.

At 7:30 a.m. the following morning, we began the long day of travel to the island. Jimson had arranged a Land Rover and driver and also hired our previous boat driver, Rae, for the seven to eight-hour boat ride in his small skiff. Because we were a small group, comprised of the three of us plus Rae and Rae's two helpers, who would also serve as guides, we had plenty of room in the boat compared to the first trip.

The outboard motor was loud and made it difficult to hear one another, so there was little conversation. Surprisingly, the ocean was gentle, unlike the rough sea I recalled from years earlier. The boat did not go slightly airborne or pound upon the water, Rae did not jerk the boat from side to side and our buttocks did not slam against the boat's hard aluminum shell. And we did not get lost or run out of fuel because Rae was better informed this time and was better prepared.

Although we looked for the village that had welcomed us when we stopped unexpectedly on our first trek, we could not find it. Rae could not recall the exact location. I was hugely disappointed, as we had brought educational materials, gifts and photos and looked forward to seeing them again. After going a good distance along the coastline to search for it, Rae turned the boat around, due to the limited petrol, and headed out to sea in search of the island.

As we neared the small island, the water became so calm that it could easily have been mistaken for a lake. I became excited at the thought of seeing our friends again and also collecting more plant specimens, especially one. This particular leaf was most important because it had early indications that it could possibly be a treatment for stroke and/or heart complications like arrhythmias.

The island was just as I remembered. Dugout canoes dotted the shoreline underneath large trees whose limbs cast their shadows beneath. As we neared the shore, several people walked out to the water's edge. I recognized many familiar faces including that of Lucas, the caretaker of the village's guest house. We waved to each other and, reaching the shallow waters, Eduardo and I jumped over

Chapter Nineteen

the sides of the skiff to greet everyone. There were handshakes and hugs ... and combinations thereof.

Handshakes began like a handshake in the United States with outstretched arms and right hands interlocking. However, in areas of Papua New Guinea, before the two shaking hands separated, often they would grab each other's index finger, steadily pulling it until they reached the tip of the finger. As the index fingers were completely released and the hands disengaged, a popping sound was made by snapping the fingers. For some reason, I could never make the popping sound like they did. Instead of one smooth motion, I would shake hands and then try to quickly snap my fingers, which made them laugh loudly.

Inviting us to stay once again at the guest house, Lucas left quickly to prepare it while we unloaded the boat. Although it had been a gorgeous day, the travel and the direct sun had drained us.

While Eduardo and I placed our bags inside the guesthouse, two young men stopped by to say that they were going to the sea to catch food for our evening meal. Recognizing one of them, who was named Gonnes, Eduardo and I walked over, shook hands and hugged. Gonnes had been one of our island guides on the first trip and was eager to join us again. We were both honored and thrilled.

The guest house was a basic wooden structure with two empty rooms, raised six feet above the ground. In the room to the right, I squatted beside my two North Face duffle bags and began to unpack their contents. Unrolling my sleeping pad, I placed it in the center of the room. Eduardo came over from his room a few feet away and helped me to hang my mosquito net above, which I

And the Silent Spoke

left bundled. As I sat in the center of the sleeping pad, I unpacked and organized the multitude of dry bags. The bags were a broad range of sizes and colors: small, medium, large and extra-large . . . orange, blue, green, yellow, red and white.

To my left I placed the bags of clothes, toiletries, pens and notebooks and my boots. To my right were bags of snacks and food as well as the EpiPens and medical kits. At the foot of my sleeping pad were cameras, batteries, an extra headlamp and flashlight, machete, Swiss Army knife and other technical odds and ends. And at the head of the pad were cutting shears, collection bags, markers and gloves, gifts for the healers as well as photos that had been taken on the first trip.

Eventually I stretched out on the mat and closed my eyes. Perspiration dripped down my face and neck and slid off my body, creating small pools of water underneath me. With a mosquito squealing in my ear, I untied the mosquito netting above and tucked the edges under the four corners of the sleeping pad. The netting immediately blocked the small amount of air that had been flowing into the room. Taking off my shirt and shorts provided little relief.

Almost an hour later, Jimson walked over to the guest house and announced that dinner had arrived. Putting the damp clothes back on my saturated body, I grabbed my headlamp and walked toward a group of men who had gathered at the water's edge around one of the dugouts. Inside the canoe were two large lobsters and an assortment of fish, including several that were a beautiful color combination of bright yellow and blue. Taking large leaves, the men wrapped the catch and walked over to place them over a small fire. There was no added salt, pepper, or any other spice. And it wasn't necessary. It was delicious.

Chapter Nineteen

After finishing the meal, Jimson, Eduardo and I continued to talk with Lucas, Gonnes and the other men until it was time to bed down for the night. The evening sounds were extraordinary, as insects and frogs chimed with the softly crashing waves.

I quickly fell asleep.

After a breakfast of ramen noodles and my favorite chicken-flavored crackers, Lucas, Jimson, Gonnes, Eduardo and I were off to search for the healers. Beside the guest house was a path that led to the center of the village. It was also the path we used on the previous trip to walk to the home of one of the healers. With day packs, collection bags and equipment, we followed the weaving path in and around trees and vegetation.

Children ran all around us and their numbers seemed to grow with each passing minute. Several of them had been playing on the ground along the path and upon seeing us, quickly got up and ran to us. Their hands, legs and bare brown bottoms were covered in white sand.

Walking further, with our eyes on the ground ahead of us, several other children caught us off guard with their giggles from above, where they straddled tree limbs under which we walked. Before long, a group of ten to fifteen children accompanied us along the path.

Almost a mile into our walk, we saw in the distance a man waving as he walked toward us. I soon realized it was Kupsey, the first healer we had met years earlier and with whom we had spent many hours. We immediately embraced and with Jimson translating, chatted a few minutes before he led us to his hut.

"I heard of your arrival," he excitedly relayed in Tok Pisin to Jimson. "I have been waiting on you. I knew that you would one day return. I knew it!"

He had aged a bit and developed a slight stoop in his stature. His salt and pepper hair had turned predominantly white. His smile, though, was exactly as I remembered . . . maybe even more beautiful.

With Jimson translating the Tok Pisin to English, we talked as we walked. Arriving at his home, we sat on a log underneath the branches of a tree. Its shade was a welcomed relief from the ninety-degree day. Even with a frequent breeze, sweat dripped down my shirt, causing the fabric to cling tightly to my skin.

For more than an hour, we talked about the island, his life and family. Speaking of his wife and children, he called for them and then proudly reintroduced each one. I then shared photos that were taken during our initial visit that I had brought for Kupsey. His wife and the four children gathered behind us, pressing up against us as they hovered over our shoulders looking at the photos. Laughing.

Pulling out the cameras, Eduardo took more photos, including many of Kupsey with his family. Afterwards, Kupsey sent the children away to play.

I shared with Kupsey our interest in additional collections of the plants that he had described to us on our first visit. With his continued permission, we would then work with researchers to further study them. Kupsey was thrilled and said that he was happy to work together and happy for our friendship, adding that he hoped that his treatments and the treatments of his village would one day help many people all over the world.

I described the plants and the treatments he had spoken of years earlier. Treatments for cough and sickness, lung problems and blood flow. Nodding, he stated that he continued to use most of them.

To make sure that I had documented the information correctly and also to remind Kupsey of the plants we had discussed years

Chapter Nineteen

earlier, I started by giving the name of the first one on my list, a tree that we had flagged as potentially beneficial for stroke or cardiovascular disease. His brow creased as he listened intently. After I recited the notes I had taken and Jimson had translated, Kupsey stared at Jimson for a few moments before looking back at me.

Hesitantly, he spoke and Jimson relayed, "He says he cleared that area last year and chopped down all the trees, including that one. They used it for firewood."

My eyes glazed over while my thoughts swirled. A deep sickening feeling hit the core of my stomach.

There were many things I had worried about with this trip back to the island. I had worried that we would not be able to find a boat driver who knew of the island and could get us there. I worried that Kupsey might not be alive, as the average life span in Papua New Guinea was fifty to sixty-five years, which I knew he was beyond. And I worried that he had not shared his knowledge with anyone else in the village and in the event of his death, the information had also perished.

But not once had I ever worried or even imagined that the trees and plants themselves would no longer be there.

Looking up at Kupsey, I asked, "Are there any other trees like it on the island?"

After pausing for a minute, he stood and motioned for us to follow. Making his own path through the forest, we walked closely behind him, stepping over fallen trees, ducking under low hanging branches while shoving others to the side. After almost an hour, he stopped at the base of a tree, looked up and patted the tree's trunk. It was about the same size as the original tree I had documented in my notes. I smiled as I looked closely at the leaves, confirming what I believed to be the same tree I had been trying to describe.

Kupsey then gestured for one of the young boys who had been following us to come to him. Speaking a dialect of Tok Pisin, he handed the young boy his machete. The boy walked to the base of the tree and placed the machete sideways in his mouth, clenching the center section with his teeth. Holding the machete in his mouth, he scampered up the tree using his bare feet to grab the bark while his arms seemed to hug the trunk. As he moved up the tree, he stopped often to slap his legs, arms, neck and face as if mosquitoes were biting him. He continued climbing until he reached a large limb directly above us. Lying flat on his stomach on top of the branch, he crawled along the branch a few feet before taking the machete out of his mouth and hacking through the limb.

Within minutes, the branch fell and with it, hundreds, if not thousands, of ants. They scattered wildly, crawling over the vegetation and anything in their path. Including us. Their mandibles sank into our flesh, which made us wince and softly groan. I stepped nearer to the tree to take a closer look at the trunk and its limbs above me, only to see that they were covered with thousands of ants. Camouflaged against the bark, they scurried across every leaf, stem and branch. Although the young boy who had climbed the tree never moaned, complained or even said a word, his body must have been covered by the insects.

It was an amazing symbiotic relationship. The ants and the tree lived as one. The tree provided sustenance and refuge for the ants, and the ants in turn provided for and protected the tree. I knew, too, that there was much more to this relationship than I could imagine.

Kupsey quickly told us that if you kill one ant, a message is sent to all the others to 'attack.' He also said that they bite and keep biting, so that you have to actually pull them off. Walking several feet away from the tree and its fallen limb, we continued to talk as

Chapter Nineteen

Kupsey brushed the ants off of my face and arms. And I did the same for him. The ants, none-the-less, continued to pierce the skin of our feet and ankles, legs and backs, arms and necks.

Under Kupsey's guidance and instruction, several young boys helped us to collect the leaves and other parts of the branch while the ants continued their assault. When the collection was completed, we walked back to Kupsey's hut where we spent two more hours with him before heading back to the guest house. In front of the guest house, I spread the leaves, twigs and wooden pieces out on woven mats to dry in the sun.

And then I joined Eduardo in the sea to wash off the ant bodies and to heal the skin.

The next day, we went in search of Nizax, the second healer, who lived on the other side of the island. Following Lucas, the guest house caretaker, we veered off one path onto a much less traveled one which was difficult to follow. When we arrived at Nizax's home, the healer was nowhere to be found.

Lucas had heard from one of the fishermen that Nizax had left the island weeks earlier to visit family on another island, but the fisherman thought that the healer would have returned by now. Unfortunately, Nizax had not. And no one knew when (or if) he would return.

Unlike most places in the world, Papua New Guinea seldom had only one healer or medicine man in a village, but rather several healers, each of whom specialized in one or more treatments. Because of this, no one knew the treatment that Nizax had shared with us on our first trip. No one even recognized the name of the plant.

Reviewing my notes and photos of the plant, I visualized the open area where the plant grew, with its few scattered trees and three-foot-tall grass-like field, but I had no clue how to get there. Lucas took one of the pictures and began asking several villagers for help. Finally, a young man replied that he knew the plant and had even seen his friend, Nizax, collect it.

The young man led us through the woods for almost an hour. The trail was barely visible due to the magnificent, dense ferns that seemed to not only drape over the path but consume it. The area was quiet and peaceful, and I became so captivated by the numerous butterflies and birds flying around us that for a moment, I forgot what we were doing.

The young man slowed when the woods and vegetation thinned. In the distance, I could see the open field-like area that I remembered. Reaching its edge, the young man bent down, pulled up several stems of the plant and, smiling, held them out for me to see. It was indeed the same plant. Looking out across the field, bundles of the long-stemmed plants with their short, narrow green leaves moved in unison almost as if they were waving in the wind.

Along with the young man, Eduardo, Jimson, Lucas, Gonnes and me, our group also included eight young children from the village. Eager to help, they ran into the surrounding area and began to pull the plants just like the young man had done. They grabbed as many as possible in their tiny hands and ran back to place the plants in our bags.

On the ground behind them lay trails of pulled plants that had slipped through their fingers. As they continued to pull the slender plants from the ground, I gathered those that fell behind.

Chapter Nineteen

Watching the children made me laugh, especially one young boy who was maybe four years old. Using both hands to pull the plants didn't leave a hand to hold up his pants. The pants, which were several sizes too big, fell to his ankles as he ran, leaving his bare bottom exposed. With both fists full, he ran, stumbled and tripped until he placed the plants inside one of the bags. Laughing, he then squatted, pulled up his pants and ran to do it all over again. I looked for a piece of string or rope to tie the pants around his waist but did not have one.

The adult villagers, on the other hand, were perplexed with our interest in the plant. To everyone other than the healer and the young man who showed us the plant, it had no value and was considered a weed. For us, the plant had indications that it could possibly be active against diabetes.

When we arrived back to the guest house, I spread the plants out in the sun to dry next to the others. Periodically, I turned them over to help ensure that both sides were dried as evenly as possible. In the evenings, the plants were placed into bags overnight to protect them from collecting dew, being blown by heavy winds in the event of an unexpected storm or walked on or scattered by someone or some creature in the dark. It was a process that I repeated each day until either they were dry, or it was time to depart.

When the last day came, it was hard to leave, as I loved the island, the healers and the people. We would have stayed several more days, but in order to have time in Jimson's village, we had to follow the itinerary we had set. After loading the boat, Eduardo, Jimson, Rae and I boarded while Rae's assistants, Lucas, Gonnes, and several other men pushed the skiff further into the water.

Many of the children also helped. They stood with bare feet at the bow, their hands against the hull as their bodies leaned into the boat. While they pushed, I reached over the side of the boat and grabbed their small hands, causing them to burst into laughter.

As we motored away, the children stood with the adults along the shoreline and waved. Waving back, we yelled in Tok Pisin, *"Tenkyu tru,"* which meant 'Thank you.'

Far to the right of where they stood, hidden from the crowd, was Kupsey. He stood alone in two feet of water. As I smiled and waved to him and he to me, tears began to form in my eyes.

He knew that we would come back.

I prayed that it would not be long before we would once again return. And when we did, that I would be able to see that smile . . . and embrace my friend once more.

Chapter Twenty

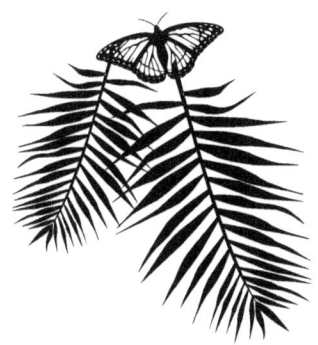

The boat ride back to Lae was uneventful and quiet. Eduardo and I reclined on top of the mound of dry bags and equipment and closed our eyes. In the back of the boat, close to Rae, sat his two assistants as well as Jimson and two villagers from the island who wanted a ride to the city. Although the pounding of the waves made it impossible to sleep, it was still rather relaxing. Every hour or so, we splashed salt water on our faces and bodies to cool off and occasionally reapplied sunscreen to help prevent the burning of our lighter flesh. The sun was intense, and there was not one cloud in the sky.

We had scheduled two days in Lae upon our return. This gave time to reorganize for the second part of the trek, to recharge batteries and for me to obtain a phytosanitary permit and to prepare the plants for shipment back to the U.S.

As a test, I shipped a small box of plants back to the lab in North Carolina with all the appropriate paperwork and permits to make sure there were no problems with customs. If everything went well, upon our return from the second part of the trek, I would ship out the remaining plants.

On the morning of the third day, Eduardo, Jimson and I negotiated a price to rent an old white Toyota Land Cruiser from a local business man. With Jimson driving, we departed the city for his family village.

It would be a full day of travel by SUV. Two young guides, lean and fit, sat next to Jimson in the front of the vehicle. In the back, Eduardo and I reclined on the two bench seats, which ran parallel to the vehicle's side windows. On the floor between us was a pile of gear, bags and supplies.

My emotions continued to be mixed over this 'replacement' region. I persisted in second guessing the decision to travel to Jimson's family village instead of going to the originally scheduled region. And I continued to battle my feelings of failure and inadequacy for not collecting the plant that could possibly prove beneficial to our researcher in the fight against cancer.

At the same time, I was excited about meeting Jimson's family and exploring the new area in the western part of the Morobe Province. The community, Jimson claimed, was eager for our arrival, for we would be the first outsiders ever invited into their village.

The journey to the village took almost nine hours. Thankfully we were in the dry season. Travel during the rainy season was restricted due to the rising waters of the Markham River, which made parts of the road impassable.

When we were a little over two hours away from the village, we left the primary road and veered onto a rarely-traveled, secondary, grassy dirt road. The road twisted and turned as it followed alongside magnificent mountains, requiring Jimson to shift the vehicle

Chapter Twenty

into four-wheel drive. The four-wheel drive also made it easy to cross several small streams.

After a while, however, we neared our greatest challenge—crossing the two-thousand-foot-wide Markham River. Approaching the river's bank, Jimson stopped the vehicle so that both guides could get out and evaluate the path we needed to take in crossing the river.

Jimson explained that the river was swift, and sections were deep. If we didn't cross at the right points, the SUV could be swept away. We watched as the guides went into the river until the water was waist deep, and often chest deep. With the water's current beating against their bodies, they stumbled and fell, struggled for footing and were frequently swept several feet downstream before regaining control.

Wanting to get a better view, Eduardo and I exited the vehicle through the rear double doors and walked around to the front of the vehicle, where we climbed into the front compartment and sat close to Jimson. Staring ahead, we watched the guides use their bodies as markers in the river. One stood closer to the northern bank while the other struggled to cross the deeper waters to get near the southern bank.

In position, they each stood in three to four feet of water and pointed from one side of the river to the other, outlining the curvy route that Jimson needed to follow. Firmly, they warned of the sections to avoid—areas that had sudden drops in depth or where the current was too swift.

At their signal, Jimson revved the engine and cautioned us to hang on tight. Putting the vehicle in first gear, he pushed the pedal to the floor before quickly shifting into second. We hit the water hard and immediately began being pulled downstream. The vehicle rocked, jolting us in all directions. Jimson accelerated by the first young man before the front of the vehicle hit the deeper, faster-flowing water, forcing him to struggle to keep the vehicle from being pulled downstream while battling to keep the SUV on course.

Several times our bodies were thrown into the air and knocked from side to side, causing Jimson to momentarily lose his grip and control of the steering wheel. Adding to the difficulty of navigating against the strong current was the rocky river bed. At the deepest point, the front of the vehicle became completely submerged, sending waves of water over the hood into the windshield. At times, the water took complete control of the vehicle, with us in it. In my mind, I waited for Eduardo to exit through his passenger window and Jimson through the driver's window, planning to follow right behind one of them. I feared if we waited too long, the vehicle would flip. But it did not.

Reaching the other side, we yelled with excitement. Behind us, with their arms swinging as they tried to run in the water, the two young men laughed and yelled back. Once on dry land, each of them gave us high fives. While the young men grabbed other clothing and changed into dry t-shirts and shorts, Eduardo and I continued to complement Jimson, who was standing next to the river, marveling at the crossing we had just made.

The road from that point on became more erratic and bumpy due to the rocky terrain. Jimson struggled to keep the vehicle on the path as the Land Cruiser barreled over small boulders and seemed to jump sideways one minute and forward the next.

When we reached the higher elevations, the road weaved in and around mountainsides, following a path created from ledges chiseled out of the mountainsides. It was uneven, rocky, and barely wide enough for two vehicles to narrowly pass. Fortunately, with only a couple of vehicles in the region, such a meeting was unlikely.

Chapter Twenty

To our left was a steep drop off, and far below flowed the Markham River.

A little less than a mile from the village, members of Jimson's community, who had been waiting for hours, gathered to welcome us. They were young and old, male and female, and they dressed in attire that was reserved for ceremonies and special occasions. Jimson explained that our arrival was a special celebration, as it would be the first time they had had outsiders stay in the village.

Young girls wore grass skirts while young boys wore sashes of green plants across their chests. Their faces were painted yellow and red, the traditional markings of the tribe. Men wore strings of small white cowry shells that were draped diagonally over their chests. Across their bodies, they strapped white, black, and pink woven satchels.

Two male elders had whole, lifeless bodies of birds-of-paradise strapped to their foreheads, their feathers magnificent combinations of blue and red.

As we greeted the chief and elders with handshakes and brief hugs (which was more our custom than theirs), garlands of pink pastel flowers were placed around our necks by several women. The chief then turned to lead us into the village. As he did so, he and several of the elders began to sing. Strapped across their chests and resting against their hips were hour-glass-shaped wooden drums. With drumheads covered in snake skins, they beat the slender two-foot-long instruments in unison.

Everyone joined in the singing and in the procession as we followed the chief down a path overgrown with tall grass and shrubs.

With small bundles of cut palm branches in each hand, the women sang as they shook the branches along with the beat of the drums, adding a swishing sound to the music.

Fifteen minutes later, we came to a clearing that was forty-by-fifty feet. The smooth dirt surface was dotted only by a few trees with the largest one standing in the center. Surrounding the area on three sides was forest. On the fourth and left side, four huts had been erected.

Jimson leaned toward us and said, "This is where we gather. Here, we have celebrations, ceremonies and discussions."

As Jimson spoke, the elders walked to the center of the cleared area and stopped in the middle, next to the large tree. Its trunk, several feet in diameter, supported numerous large branches that extended outward fifteen feet and more, providing an area of shade for the elders. Turning around, they faced the three of us and, in a semi-circle, sat on the ground in front of the tree. Other villagers walked by us and quietly gathered behind the elders, while other members of the tribe emerged from the surrounding woods.

Close to one hundred and fifty people stood several rows deep in a large semi-circle, ten feet beyond where the elders sat. Once everyone settled, Jimson spoke to the chief, elders and village in Tok Pisin. After a few minutes, he said, "I told them that you are the friends I have talked about. That you have traveled many miles and across the ocean in order to visit our village. And that you are interested in the plants we use for medicine."

Jimson then looked directly at me and said, "Amy, you can now address the chief, elders and village."

With Jimson translating, I acknowledged and greeted first the chief and elders and then the village before stating how honored we were to meet them and to be in their beautiful village. I thanked them

Chapter Twenty

for the privilege and for the wonderful reception, which touched our hearts. I continued by introducing Eduardo and myself and describing the work we were doing and our interest in visiting their village. I spoke at length, detailing how we had worked with other villages to collect and analyze plants and natural remedies in hopes of helping others to benefit also from their powerful medicines.

I stated that with their permission, we could also film and share their lives and their village with many children all over the United States and world, explaining that we had worked with Jimson in other regions of the country and that we would like the opportunity to explore a relationship with them.

After I finished, the chief and then each elder spoke, one after another, expressing gratitude that we were visiting their village. They asked where we lived in the United States and how long it had taken us to travel to their country. And what was it like to be in a plane and like a bird in the air. They asked about our families, our parents and siblings . . . and if we had children. They asked about televisions. And if we would take their picture.

They continued by saying that they had good medicine and many things to share. They were happy that we had traveled so far to see them because they wanted to have opportunities for development—opportunities that they had heard had been given to other villages. Development was good and it brought money to have things like better clothes and shoes, tools and even a vehicle that the village could use to go to market or transport someone to a doctor if they were sick or badly hurt.

After the elders spoke, the villagers who had gathered around them were also given the opportunity to speak. Several men and women expressed similar sentiments as those of the elders, almost verbatim, until everyone who wished to speak had spoken.

I then asked about the needs of the village and what we could do for them. For a few minutes, the elders leaned forward toward one another and quietly spoke before turning back toward us and responding. Clearing his throat, the chief began to describe the village's two greatest needs: education and a medical clinic for emergencies and for the things that they were unable to treat.

As the chief elaborated, Jimson translated. "The children must walk seven hours to the school. There, they stay all week until it is time for them to walk the seven hours home. It is most difficult for the little ones to leave their mothers and be away for so many days at a time. The older children care for the younger ones as well as themselves—preparing food each day, washing and dressing themselves and the younger ones and tending to the assignments from their teachers.

The closest medical clinic is eighteen miles away. When someone is terribly hurt or very sick, it is difficult to transport them over such a distance. In the rainy season, it takes even longer and is more difficult as the river is too dangerous to cross near us, so we must go several miles farther to get to a bridge to cross. If there is no vehicle, we must carry the person, including across the river, which is most difficult and dangerous where the water is deep."

When he finished, the chief and the elders stood while several women stepped in front of them and placed woven mats on the ground for them to sit upon, maintaining the semi-circle. Three additional mats were placed directly across from the chief, making the circle complete. On these three mats, Eduardo, Jimson and I were motioned to sit. Surprisingly, the thinly woven, flat green mats were soft and comfortable.

A young man then stepped between two of the elders and positioned two large palm leaves in the middle of the circle, end to end and slightly overlapping. Next, he spread smaller leaves on

Chapter Twenty

the ground in front of each person in the circle. Afterwards, two women stepped into the circle and placed two black clay bowls on top of the larger palm leaves.

Within the first bowl, Jimson explained, were small bananas cooked in coconut milk. In the second one, small chunks of pig cooked with ginger.

Beside the clay bowls, the women placed several thin, shaved sticks, five inches long. With pointed ends, they looked like chopsticks, but instead of using two of them to pick up food, only one was used, to spear the food. Following the actions of the elders, Eduardo and I pierced food in both containers and placed it on the smaller leaves in front of us, using the leaves much like plates. The meat was juicy and tender and the combined flavors of the two dishes were a culinary masterpiece. It was so yummy, I could have eaten much more, but I only had a few bites as we knew that this food, especially a pig, was a rare treat and anything not eaten by those in the circle would be shared with the others in the village.

As we ate and talked about hunting and cooking, short blasts of air hit the back of my neck, forearms and crossed legs. The sudden breezes were refreshing. And yet highly unusual. Looking behind me, I noticed several women standing directly behind Eduardo and me waving palm branches to shoo away the many flies, who also found the food delightful. I smiled and thanked them.

Moments later, the chief's daughter brought over a coconut with its top chopped off and handed it to me to drink. Smiling, I handed it back for her to drink first. Although she seemed to be caught off-guard, she grinned and took a small sip. The elders and villagers laughed. After taking another sip, she handed it back to me.

The coconut water was sweet, cool and refreshing. After two sips, I handed it to the elder to my right, something that Jimson whispered to me to do. After the elder drank from it, he passed it to the elder to his right, and so on until everyone had taken a drink. Another coconut was then brought to Eduardo, who took two sips and then passed it to his right until it went around the circle as well.

For several days, we stayed within the village and spent time with the chief, elders and villagers. Jimson, Eduardo and I also ventured out of the village with one of the oldest elders to explore the surrounding forests, which contained many of the remedies used by the village.

One afternoon, we walked for a couple of hours until we reached an open area about the size of a football field that was overgrown with a grass-like vegetation, three to four feet tall. Protruding from the center of the field, was one tree. The elder made a path to the tree and without hesitating, began chopping off several pieces of its thick, white bark. With the pieces gathered in his left hand, he took one fragment and held it in the air with his right hand, describing the bark as a treatment for one of the two most deadly snake bites in the region.

Jimson translated, "If the snake bites, a person must quickly get the bark—or he will die. If it is longer than one hour before he gets the medicine, he will not live."

"What does the snake look like?" I asked. "Where does it live?"

"It is black and white," Jimson replied. Then, extending his right arm and making a large swooping gesture from left to right, he responded, "The snake lives here."

Later, back in the U.S., I wondered if the snake was the feared Papuan taipan, one of the most venomous snakes in the world.

The elder led us out of the grassy field and back through the forest until he stopped at another tree. The tree had striking features, not only with its trunk which was five-feet-wide, but with its gnarly roots, partially above ground, stretching away from the trunk much like the tentacles of an octopus. The tree's sap, he explained, was used to treat a woman's sore breasts during breast feeding. The sap would also heal the baby's lips and mouth if there was any kind of irritation.

A few feet away from this tree, he pointed to a low-lying green plant. The plant, he stated casually, was boiled in water and then sipped as a tea to cure fatigue and sore muscles.

On the fourth day, we took the SUV and traveled with the chief to explore an area of their land that was located several miles away. On the way back to the village, Jimson noticed a large black cloud forming across the sky in the distance. Stopping, he put the vehicle in park, turned off the ignition and asked that we get out to take a closer look. The cloud was moving quickly toward us and its shape was constantly changing. Like a large amoeba, its edges undulated as they enlarged one minute and contracted the next; yet the mass also swirled, flowing first in one direction and then another, constantly maintaining a fluid-like state.

As we stared into the sky, I wondered if it was a severe weather phenomenon, like a tornado—and if we might need to retreat in the opposite direction. But before I could ask any questions, Jimson announced that it was a large roost of flying foxes. They were not actual foxes, but very big bats. Later I would learn that they were some of the largest in the world and belonged to the genus Pteropus.

Jimson then asked us to hurry and get back into the SUV, and he would try to follow them until they landed. He explained that the roost would find a large, wooded area in which to land, and if we would like to see them up close, he would try to find them. Giddy, we quickly got in, slammed the doors shut and, sitting on the front edges of our seats, peered into the distant sky.

I couldn't help but to think of all the episodes of Mutual of Omaha's Wild Kingdom with Marlin Perkins and Jim Fowler that I had watched as a child. Many times in my childhood, and admittedly even into adulthood, I had imagined being on location for such a wildlife documentary program.

As we got closer to the bats, we could see the shadow on the land beneath them, cast by their bodies much like the shadows cast by clouds. Because the road we were traveling was enveloped by tall trees, Jimson frequently lost sight of the roost and was forced to stop the vehicle, turn off the engine and listen for their caws.

At the crest of a mountain, with an expansive view of the surrounding area, we finally found their perch. Standing outside the vehicle, we stared at what must have been thousands of the bats swarming a section of swampy forest in the near distance. Getting back into the vehicle, Jimson followed the road only a few minutes before he veered off the road, weaved in and around foliage and eventually stopped at the edge of the swamp.

The noise was loud and intense. High-pitched squawks and squeals drowned out every other sound, making it difficult to hear each other without screaming. Eduardo and I climbed and stood on top of the SUV, watching as hundreds of dark brown bodies darted through the wetland, swarming the sky above and around us before nestling within the swath of trees.

It was mesmerizing and yet eerie, and although it brought back memories of Alfred Hitchcock's *The Birds*, it was not frightening.

As we watched the creatures flying above, Jimson whistled loud enough to get our attention and motioned for us to come to him. Emerging from the swamp behind him was a young man, wet from his thighs down to his bare feet. In his right hand, he held a two-inch-round wooden stick, and in his left hand, he gripped the legs of several bats, which dangled lifelessly.

Chapter Twenty

A handsome young man with thick, black hair in his mid- to late-twenties, he wore a pair of faded, ragged shorts and a torn gray shirt. After introductions, I couldn't help but stare at the wooden club and then, the creatures, which he proudly raised high.

It was difficult to look at the poor beings, some still barely alive.

Dropping the bats on the ground, he squatted and meticulously went through the pile of bodies, tossing several to the side before picking one up. As he stood, he grabbed the ends of both its wings, stretching the appendages as much as possible to reveal a three-foot wingspan. While he did so, Jimson explained that the bats were food for his family.

Later, when we were back in the vehicle, Jimson told us that only men who were bad hunters killed bats. He would never provide such food for his family because good hunters didn't feed their families such things.

Back in the village, the women were eager to share their customs and traditions, which included the tattoo markings on their faces and bodies. The markings were specific for their tribe and had been used for generations. As I sat with a group of women in a circle on the ground, Jimson squatted behind me and translated.

"We take a sharp thorn or sharp object and make many small holes in the skin," Jimson described as the chief's daughter spoke. "You must do it quickly and push hard so that there is blood. When the holes bleed, we cover them with burned firewood. Charcoal.

The charcoal must get inside each hole because that is what makes the markings black. The markings will fade, so you must do it again when it becomes hard to see."

She then announced that the next time I came to the village, they would give me the markings too.

I imagined returning home with the three parallel black lines across my white cheeks. And then pondered how I would try to explain it to my partner and parents.

Three times since our arrival to his village, Jimson mentioned a virgin forest that remained largely untouched by man because of its location. Walking, it would take a couple of days for a person to reach the area. By SUV, it would take up to five hours, depending on rain, going slowly and crossing multiple streams.

Although he had not seen the land in many years, he was excited to show it to us, as it was also home to many exotic birds, like the birds-of-paradise. Of the forty-three species known in the world, thirty-eight species lived in Papua New Guinea.

So on our fifth and final day in Jimson's village, we loaded the SUV early in the morning before sunrise to travel northwest to the virgin forest. As soon as we were on our way, Jimson announced that he had news for us.

"Word of your arrival has spread quickly." Jimson said. "Hours after you went to bed last night, a young boy arrived in the village with a message from his grandfather—a healer. His grandfather is an old man, and he wants to meet you. He sent his grandson to request you visit him. He wants to share his medicine with you."

After a brief pause, Jimson continued, "His home is near the virgin forest. If you would like to visit him, I suggest we spend only two or three hours in the forest, that way, we will have time to visit the elder."

Chapter Twenty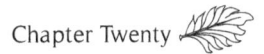

"Absolutely," I responded. "Wow. This is great."

First, we would see the virgin forest and second, visit the healer. Because it had been many years since Jimson had been to the forest, we hired Baia, a young man from a nearby village, to drive the SUV and serve as our guide.

The drive was peaceful and quiet. It was early morning and dark, and I, for one, remained half asleep. With the windows down, we hoped to glimpse an exotic bird, mammal or even snake in the misty terrain. But with dim headlights and with little illumination, it was difficult to distinguish a cluster of foliage from an animal . . . or a vine from a snake.

We rode in silence and listened to the sounds of birds and insects announcing the new dawn. Three hours into the drive, however, we passed through a small village. A handful of huts lined the road, several of which belonged to some of Baia's friends. Noticing a friend outside one of the huts near a fire, Baia tooted the horn and stopped for a moment to introduce us and chat before continuing the drive.

Even though we failed to see any of the colorful exotic birds that morning, the virgin forest was spectacular. Jimson did not know the healing plants well, but he knew of a few. The ones he pointed out, however, also happened to be the same plants that the elder had shown to us in the days prior.

The forest, however, was pristine. It smelled clean, yet musky and woodsy, like the aroma of decomposing wood. It was quiet except for the songs of birds and the clicking, chirping sounds made by insects. A large creek flowed through the section we explored and was surrounded on either side by waist-high ferns. Beyond the ferns, magnificent old hardwoods created such a thick canopy above that it was almost impossible to see the sky.

We returned to the SUV a couple of hours later, heading back in the direction we had come with plans to spend time with the healer in his village. Along the way, we once again drove through the small village where we had met Baia's friend earlier that morning. In the road ahead, she waved her arms for us to stop. As we slowed, she ran over to Baia's window and with shallow breaths explained that she had been waiting for hours for us to pass through. With tears in her eyes, she continued to tell us that there had been a horrible accident.

Trembling slightly, she spoke as Jimson translated. "A truck overturned several hours earlier on its way to the market."

Jimson explained, "The truck is only one of two in the entire area that is used to transport people to and from the market. The market is eighteen miles away from my village—and much further away for these people, and many others."

She continued and Jimson translated, "The truck was going too fast around a curve and it rolled over. Everyone was hurt. Some very badly. It is terrible."

With tears flowing and with heightened emotion, she spoke further as Jimson solemnly uttered, "They say that two people are dead. Including a child."

As in disbelief, Jimson spoke slowly and solemnly, "It was a full truck. Maybe forty to fifty people. Because it takes so long to walk to the market, people crowd in the back of the open bed truck. The truck travels the mountain pass that we had to drive after crossing the river. The cliffs are very steep. When the truck toppled, everyone was thrown out of the truck. And off the side of the mountain."

The lady spoke further, and Jimson translated, "This is very, very bad. Driving the truck was Baia's father. Baia's brother had gone to help his father that day and was sitting beside his father in

Chapter Twenty

the front seat. She does not know if they are dead or alive."

Jimson listened intently to the woman and once again began to translate her words. "She is afraid that if Baia's father and brother are alive, there will be a coup formed against them and his entire family because of the harm and deaths that his father has caused. There is already great anger."

Baia sat silent. I watched his face in the rear-view mirror. He stared ahead without expression before turning to the lady to ask three more questions. Jimson relayed. "Baia is asking if she knows if everyone has been taken to the clinic. When did the accident happen? And if she knows the names of those who died."

Jimson lowered his head and slowly shook it right to left and back again. Quietly he said, "This is very, very bad."

After a few moments, Jimson continued. "The truck stops near every village to pick up people who need to go to the market. I am afraid that my friends and family may have been in the truck too. This is terrible.

Such a thing has never happened here. He must have been driving too fast. I am afraid for Baia and worry for his father and brother. I pray they are alive. I pray, too, that my family and friends did not go to the market today."

Baia thanked the lady and then quickly accelerated. As he did so, Jimson continued, "Because the accident happened many hours earlier, she thinks most of the people have already been transported to the local clinic.

Would it be okay if we do not go to the healer's village but instead allow Baia to drive directly to the clinic?"

"Of course," Eduardo and I said in unison.

"We insist!" I added.

After a few moments of silence, Baia and Jimson spoke to one another in Tok Pisin before Jimson turned around to us. "Baia is asking if you would please help us. You are medical professionals and have knowledge that we do not. We have never had such a horrible accident and the injuries are very, very bad. The clinic is small and there is only one doctor and sometimes one nurse. There is not much medicine or supplies. They cannot handle this many people or bad injuries."

Although Baia was driving much faster, it would be another two to three hours before we reached Jimson's village and another two to three hours from his village to the clinic. Regardless, we made a plan. We would stop very quickly at Jimson's village where Eduardo and I would run to the hut and grab our additional medical kits and supplies. At the same time, Jimson would send a young boy to the healer's village where we were expected to arrive that day, with our apologies and an explanation of the situation.

It was almost an hour later when we came upon the toppled truck. A young man waved his hands and walked in the middle of the road toward our SUV until he got to Baia's window. He cautioned us to go slow and to hug the left side of the road, where he would help us pass through. He then described the incident, the toppled truck and the debris in the road. Asking him if there was anyone we could help, he stated that all the injured had been transported to the local clinic.

Baia put the vehicle in park, and the three of us got out to walk around the truck and the site of the accident. Around us, blood was splattered across dirt and rocks. Scattered articles of clothing, baskets and broken glass surrounded the truck, whose front end and right side were smashed in like a half-crumpled soda can.

My heart sank. My eyes filled with tears. I turned my head and walked away from the others, hiding my emotions. I fought hard

Chapter Twenty

to stifle the feelings erupting inside of me as I thought of the two who had lost their lives. Especially the child. I thought of those injured and imagined their cries.

I stood at the edge of the mountainside, only a few feet from the toppled vehicle . . . and looked around and down below. Forty feet ahead was a sheer drop-off down the mountainside. However, where the truck had overturned, there was a ten-foot-wide ledge, five feet down, covered in vegetation. The ledge appeared to have caught those who were thrown over the side of the mountain. Had the wreck occurred just a few feet further, the injuries and death toll would most likely have been catastrophic.

Arriving at Jimson's village, Eduardo and I jumped out of the vehicle and ran to the hut to grab the other medical kits and supplies. Word had already spread of the accident, and Jimson's family and other members of the village gathered around the SUV, crying while relaying the reports they had heard. Even though no one from Jimson's village had been in the truck, for them every village in the area was considered community. And every person, family.

As many people as possible piled into the vehicle with us to go to the clinic. The back of the SUV had two side benches which allowed four to five people to sit facing each other. On one bench sat the women and on the other, the men. The chief's wife, who sat beside me to my right, and the chief's daughter, who sat to my left, each grabbed one of my hands. We continued to hold hands for the next hour.

On the bench across from us, the chief sat next to Eduardo, resting his right arm on Eduardo's shoulders. The others in the vehicle comforted each other as well, either holding hands or having their arms around one another.

With Baia driving, the chief, and then the others, recounted the story they had heard about the accident, giving their individual editorials. For more times than either Eduardo or I could recall, they thanked us for going to help.

Even though Eduardo was a paramedic and a wilderness survival expert, and I was a pharmacist, we were not sure how much we could assist the doctor and nurse. Regardless, we would do anything and everything we possibly could. And that alone somehow brought comfort to our new friends.

It took over two hours to get from the village to the clinic. And it seemed an eternity.

On the grounds surrounding the clinic were two to three hundred people. Families, friends, community . . . supporting and praying for those who were suffering inside. Baia drove the vehicle to the front entrance and we swiftly jumped out and hurried inside the clinic. Immediately, a man took us to the one doctor, and we joined him as he went from patient to patient.

With Jimson translating, he explained, "I have never seen anything like this. We do not have the resources to handle something on this scale. As soon as I heard of the wreck, I sent word by radio to neighboring clinics and the hospital in Lae to send help immediately. But it will take another hour or so for them to get here."

Within the clinic, there were two large rooms and in each room were twenty or more patients. Each injured person had several family members and friends by their side. Some of the patients were lying on cots; others were lying on the floor. Most had cuts and gashes, and many had broken bones, including compound fractures. Upon initial evaluations, the doctor believed that two people had broken backs, several had multiple fractures and many

Chapter Twenty

with at least one broken bone, while one had a punctured lung with numerous broken ribs.

As the doctor attended to some patients, I walked with Eduardo as he helped to evaluate others.

After a while, we discussed the medicines and supplies the clinic had on hand. The doctor led us to a room where there were several shelves of pharmaceuticals, bandages and even IV fluids. The amounts, however, were minimal.

The doctor walked over to a section of the room and, with a large swooping gesture with his arm, spoke as Jimson translated, "I have no idea what the medicines in this area are for or how to administer them. No one does."

With Jimson continuing to translate, the doctor then looked at me and asked, "Can you please tell me what they are and how to use them?"

Picking up the bottles one by one, I recognized only a few. The others were in languages and under names that were foreign to me. I opened the boxes and looked for information sheets, anything that might give a clue . . . for names that might be similar to the brand or generic names, or even chemicals I recognized. But no matter how hard I looked, I failed to decipher anything on most of the bottles.

It was unreal.

There, on the shelves, were potential life-saving medications, but without the information and knowledge of what they were and how to use them, they were useless. The clinic had received them under the best intentions, but somewhere along the way, failures in communication prevented their use. Without translations, the bottles would likely continue to sit on the shelves until their expiration dates forced their destruction.

With the medications I could determine and the medications in stock that the doctor knew about and could use, the most powerful thing for pain was an equivalent to acetaminophen (Tylenol). There was nothing stronger to ease the severe pain of the many patients in agony only feet away. Nothing for the intense pain of their broken bones, nothing for nausea and vomiting . . . nothing to relax their muscles or ease their anxiety. Antibiotics and antimicrobials were few and not nearly enough for the wounds and possible infections.

Emptying our medical kits, we worked together with the doctor to quickly and carefully document each bottle, translating the words and directions both on the bottles and on paper. Making extensive notes, I went over them again with the nurse as Jimson translated. We gave everything we had that he might need: antibiotics, muscle relaxants, pain meds, meds for nausea, vomiting, anaphylaxis, fungal infections, bandages, eye washes, thermometers, wraps and so on.

We stayed for hours, until additional medical personnel arrived from nearby clinics, and the most seriously injured were transferred out to the hospital in Lae. In the process, we learned that Baia's father and brother had indeed survived. His father, however, had multiple breaks in his left leg. Like several others with broken bones, his father refused treatment by the clinic, opting instead to be treated by the local bone doctor, who followed the traditional ways of healing. The bone doctor, who Jimson said was also called the witch doctor, had healed many broken bones over many years and with great success.

The bone doctor specialized in broken bones and was said to heal them so well that a man could return to his fields with normal activity and as strong as ever. Using plants and tight bandages as

Chapter Twenty

well as intense physical manipulation, the healer realigned the bones and healed the injuries. His patients would stay in a hut close to his home so that he could constantly attend to them. The treatments often took weeks.

After we had done all that we could, we left the clinic to visit Baia's father, who was with the witch doctor. In the accident he had suffered two compound fractures in his left leg. Although I imagined he was in intense pain, he did not show it. He sat on the floor, his leg tightly bound by strips of cloth and his wife by his side. He spoke calmly as he described how the truck had flipped, causing his leg to be pinned underneath the steering wheel. Several men had helped to free him. He would remain with the bone doctor for two or three weeks, maybe longer, before he would be allowed to return to his home.

Outside the healer's hut, Baia spoke of many threatening things that were being said about his father and their family, comments by the families of those who were injured in the accident. There was much anger and blame directed toward his father, whom they believed was driving too fast and should have known better. Baia feared that his father and his family would be harmed or forced to leave the community.

Community was everything.

Members within the community were family. They took care of one another. It was the only family Baia had ever known. It was the only life Baia had ever known. But now, these members of his family were not only cursing his father and his family but also threatening to banish them.

It was the final night in Jimson's village. Before leaving, the chief asked if he could drive our SUV. I immediately said yes . . . and then realized that the chief had never driven a vehicle before.

And it was a stick shift.

With Eduardo, the chief's wife and daughter and me in the back of the vehicle, the chief started the ignition and turned on the head lights. Next to him in the passenger seat sat Jimson, who served as the driving instructor.

As Jimson directed him to slowly lift his foot off the clutch, the vehicle surged, only for the chief to suddenly slam on the brakes, bringing the vehicle to a jarring stop. Then, he repeated the process over and over again. One minute our bodies were thrust forward, the next, they came to a crashing halt.

We laughed until we cried. Jimson begged him to stop but the chief insisted that he knew how to drive. With no seat belts in the vehicle, our bodies were thrown forward and then backwards, side to side, and all we could do was roar with laughter.

The following morning, we loaded the vehicle and prepared for the drive back to Lae. Eduardo and I thanked and hugged the chief, the elders and others before getting inside the SUV. With the rear doors swung open, we sat near the back of the vehicle on the edges of the side benches saying our final farewells while the chief's wife and daughter held strong our hands as we hugged once more. It was sad to leave, and yet, every time we looked at the chief, we couldn't help but to laugh at his driving lesson. And him, with us.

On the way back, we stopped at the clinic to see if we could offer any further assistance. With everyone cared for by the recently arrived nurses and medical staff, we said our goodbyes. And began the trip back to Lae.

Chapter Twenty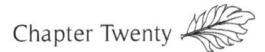

Traveling down the road, I stared out the window and recalled the events of the past twenty-four hours. And of the trip to Jimson's village.

What were the chances of such an accident happening? And to a driver who had driven the road hundreds of times before? And what were the chances that Eduardo and I would be there when it did?

What were the chances that our originally scheduled destination would be deemed too dangerous to explore and that our path would be redirected to this village . . . at this point in time?

For weeks I had been second-guessing the change in the itinerary and the redirection to Jimson's family village. I had been frustrated by our failure to collect the specimen in the mid-west region—a specimen that in years to come might possibly save lives. But I slowly began to see that we had been divinely guided away from harm and into the lives of others who needed us at that exact moment in time.

I realized, too, that we had traveled almost halfway around the world to explore indigenous medicine in efforts to bring those treatments to the rest of the world . . . only to be reminded that they also needed ours.

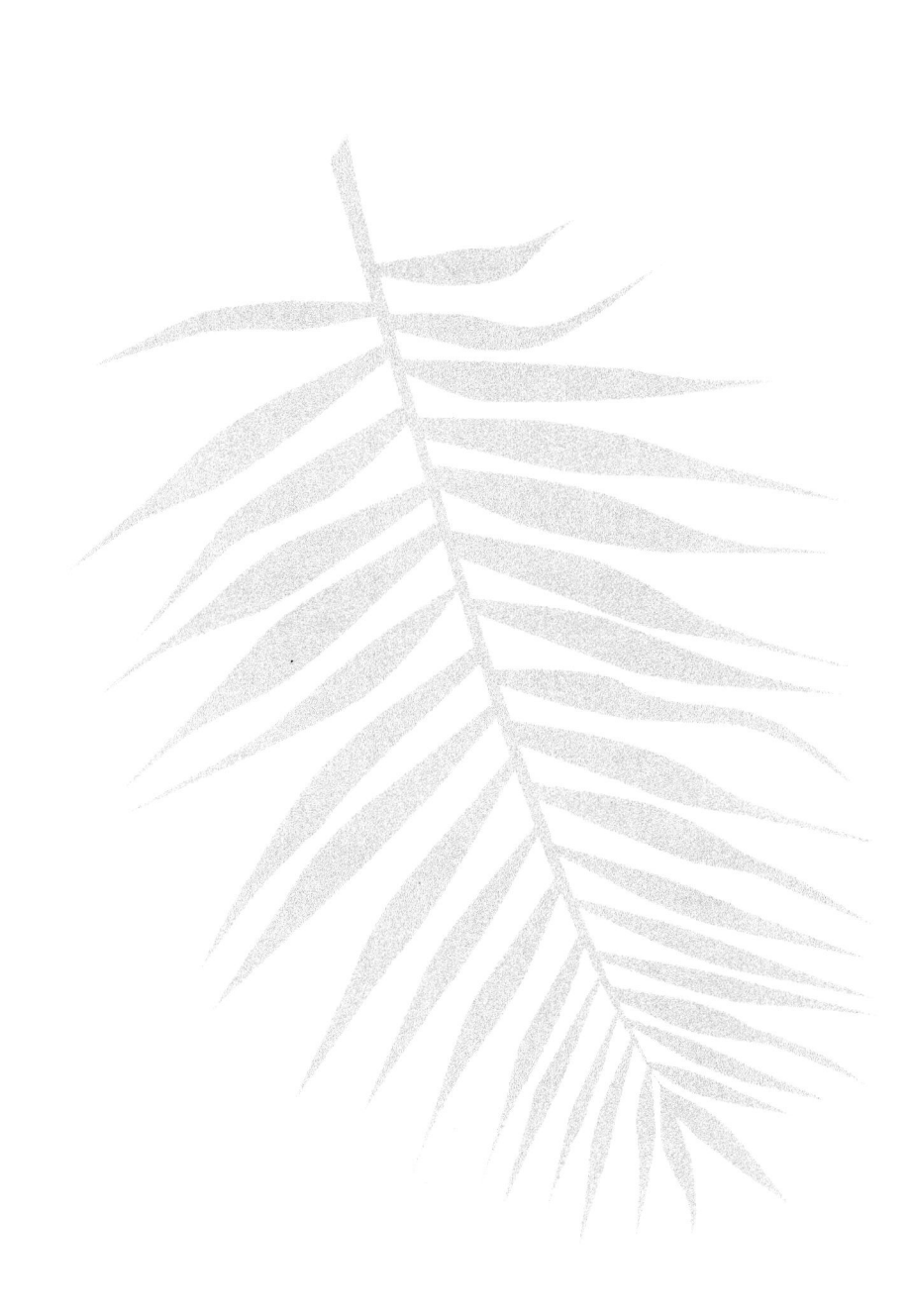

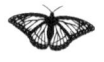
Chapter Twenty-One

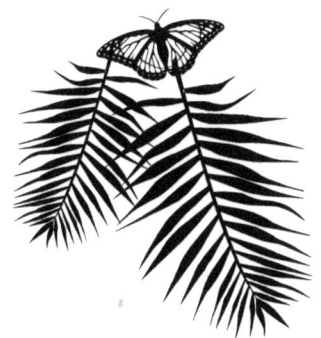

Back in Lae, I learned that the small box of plants that I had shipped eight days earlier had arrived safely in North Carolina. Following the same procedure of paperwork and permits, I then packed the remaining plants and shipped them out the following day.

The same day, Eduardo and I flew back to the capital city of Port Moresby. Two days later, we left Papua New Guinea for home.

Two weeks after my return to North Carolina, I received a message from the local UPS store in High Point, where Natural Discoveries has a mailbox, stating that the DHL package had arrived and was ready for pick up. It was the first time ever that U.S. Customs had not contacted me or our customs broker for information before clearing a package's entry. At the UPS store, a young man retrieved the box and placed it on the counter.

But something was wrong. Something was terribly wrong.

Before me was a small five-by-twelve-inch box; not the two-by-three-foot box I had personally packed to ship. Panicking, I grabbed the small box and checked the label. The correct label was on it as well as the paperwork that I had so carefully prepared to go with the packing slip on the side of the box.

The box was heavy . . . very heavy for the small amount of lightweight plants that could possibly fit inside. Although I knew that I had shipped only one large box with one label and one set of paperwork, I asked, "Are there any other boxes?"

"No," he replied. "Only one."

I walked to the car not knowing whether to scream or cry. My mind could not process what was happening. I only knew that it was not good.

If there had been a problem with U.S. Customs, they would have contacted me, and especially before destroying anything. So it must have been an issue with the shipment leaving Papua New Guinea.

Sitting in the car outside the UPS store, I used my keys and ripped through the packing tape to open the box. Inside there were no leaves, roots or bark . . . but sealed aluminum cans. They reminded me of cans of army rations, two inches in height and three inches in diameter.

On each can, scribbled with a bold black marker was a lot number, a date, and the words PACKED TUNA.

I stared at the box and its contents while tears formed in my eyes. I imagined telling Malahe, our one and only outside investor in Natural Discoveries, that the $35,000 set aside for the return trek was not only unsuccessful in collecting any new specimens, we also failed to collect the additional specimens needed to continue initial research. If the plants could not successfully be collected and recollected, the premise of the entire company was in jeopardy.

Chapter Twenty-One

Malahe had been the only one in the early stages who believed in the mission enough to financially support it. Without her investment, the research would have stopped a year earlier. And the company likely would not have survived.

The thought of failing her made me physically nauseated. To fail as a steward of her money churned my stomach inside out, while overwhelming thoughts of failure bombarded me.

I was failing our researchers by not successfully recollecting and collecting new specimens. I was failing the healers who had entrusted me with their medicines and their treatments. And I was failing my friends, family and even strangers—who were desperately longing for cures.

I sat in the car for an indeterminate amount of time and stared at the cans in my lap. My emotions were all over the place. I was furious. I was numb.

I wept.

But then something happened—something snapped deep within, urging me not to give up. I phoned DHL and begged them to find the lost shipment. I called our guide, Jimson, in Papua New Guinea and explained the situation. He was upset and yet reassuring, believing that he would call back shortly with the location of the plants. After hanging up, he returned to the local DHL office to have them search for our missing box.

Jimson and I speculated that the labels and paperwork had accidentally been switched with another shipment at the office in Papua New Guinea. Unfortunately, the DHL office provided little help, only to say that no one else had reported an error in shipment. When Jimson asked which packages were shipped right before and right after ours, which might have been accidentally mixed up with our box, they had no answer. They had a record of the packages that were shipped the same day, but they could not determine which packages were shipped around the same time.

Time became very critical and my anxiety increased with each passing hour and day. Without the appropriate paperwork and contact information attached to our box, the plants would likely be immediately rejected by a Customs official and therefore destroyed. No matter what country the box had entered.

A kind of craziness took over me as I hung on to every bit of hope that the box would be found with its contents intact. I refused to believe that they had been destroyed. I refused to give up.

Because of the fifteen-hour time difference between the United States and Papua New Guinea, Jimson and I hounded DHL around the clock. We became relentless in tracking and re-tracking every step.

My stress level was beyond anything I had ever experienced. With every possible lead, I would become excited only to then get depressed when the lead was a dead end. I was in the office at 2:00 a.m., 3:00 a.m., 4:00 a.m. almost every night talking with Jimson and various DHL employees and managers in the U.S., Papua New Guinea and globally. For two weeks I got very little sleep. And although the DHL employees were kind and sympathetic, for two weeks we had no answers.

After fifteen days, DHL discovered paperwork that led them to believe that the plants might have been sent to a company in Singapore. They discovered that a shipment to Singapore was logged in at a time that was close to when our shipment had been logged. I googled the company, called and sent emails to several people within the company.

Hours later that same evening I received a phone call. With a strong accent, the lady on the other end introduced herself as Yi Ling. She told me that she had received my email and that her company had

Chapter Twenty-One

indeed received the box of dried plants. She continued by saying that they knew that the plants were important, so they had immediately placed them in a controlled temperature environment. Elaborating, she said that as a scientist, she had worked with plants, and that the leaves in our box had dried further compared to their condition when they arrived but that they were still in very good shape.

Yi Ling stated that they had been expecting cans of tuna from a company in Papua New Guinea weeks earlier, but the shipment had been lost in transit. The cans were being shipped for analysis and testing at her company in Singapore.

As I hung up the phone, I cupped my hands to my face and cried. I didn't know whether they were tears of gratitude for Yi Ling and the company for protecting and taking such great care of our plants . . . or if they were tears of joy that our company was saved . . . or tears of relief that it was all over. I imagined it was a combination of everything.

Of all the possible destinations and of all the packages with which to have been mixed up, there could not have been a better mistake and a better caretaker. I believed that perhaps because Customs had been familiar with the large Singapore company, they had allowed the plants to transit without inspecting the contents.

In my office, I immediately scanned the necessary paperwork for Customs and emailed them to Yi Ling, who attached them to the box of plants and called DHL for pick-up. Re-labeling the box of canned tuna, I did likewise.

Yi Ling would always be considered an angel to me and our company.

She also served as a reminder to me that our research and the mission in my life continued to be divinely protected and guided in ways far beyond my comprehension. I thought about the timing and wondered what would have happened if we had shipped the box of plants at a different hour of the day or on a different day. Or if the shipment going to the Singapore company had shipped at a different time and day. I cringed at the thought.

It took almost two weeks before I received a call from U.S. Customs and then from the UPS store that a package had arrived. As I drove to pick up the box of plants, the only thing I felt was an extraordinary amount of gratitude. I didn't believe that I had been a victim or that the world had been against me. Rather, I had a strange feeling that there was something much deeper going on . . . something more important that I needed to learn.

I, however, had no idea what it could be.

At home, I carefully opened the box. Inside was the precious cargo that had been shipped almost two months earlier. One by one, I pulled out the bags of plants, closely inspecting each one before placing it on my desk in front of me.

Holding each bag, I recalled the collection of each plant and the days spent with the villages and healers. As I looked at the specimens collected during the first part of the trek, I especially recalled collecting the leaves for which the young boy had climbed the tree to cut the tree's branch. And I remembered the sound that the branch made when it hit the ground.

And then, it struck me.

The branch.

The ants.

We had not only cut off the branch, which was a part of a living organism, we had wreaked havoc on countless life forms that

Chapter Twenty-One

depended upon it. The tree was alive, and its limbs were a part of it just like arms and legs are parts of the human body.

All over the world, trees were constantly fallen, especially in the name of progress. The demise of each, however, also resulted in turmoil, death and devastation for many countless species of life. Although our actions of collecting medicinal plants were intended to utilize natural resources for the betterment of mankind, we had nonetheless failed to deeply honor and respect the entities and organisms whose lives we had impacted.

The plants, trees and organisms were not just specimens; they were first and foremost gifts from God. They were vital for the delicate balance of the earth's ecosystem. For mankind, they also became the materials for buildings and huts, paper and clothes, food and medicine, bowls and boats. They provided nutrients and sustenance, safety and protection.

Their contributions and value to our planet were beyond comprehension.

Attempting to understand nature by focusing on identifications, classifications and categorizations, testings and analyses had limited my vision and perspective of the fullness and reality of life. Just as important, or perhaps even more so, were the symbiotic relationships and the energetic worlds, interchanges and interactions that we had yet to fully tap and understand.

For me to have continued with such a myopic view would have been a tragedy, for I would have failed to glimpse the true grandeur of life.

Different philosophies battled within me, for I believed that nature could, and would, heal the world in many ways. And science, working with nature, could and would bring a plethora of medical treatments to the world. Finding a balance between the two worlds, however, would take a lifetime.

Mother Nature awakened yet another realm within me as she continued nurturing the idealist in me and prodding my curiosity. I thought more deeply about the interactions and interconnectivity between and amongst plants, insects, animals and microbes, combined with the nutrients from the rain, sun and soil.

She beckoned me to look deeper, challenging what I believed to be true. And to search not only for the significance and value of an individual organism, but to recognize and honor its contributions to the whole.

She encouraged me to embrace change . . . and fear stagnation.

But perhaps most of all, Mother Nature further enticed the explorer in me. And as I continued to map the course upon which I would walk, she held my hand. And whispered to my soul.

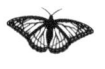
Chapter Twenty-Two

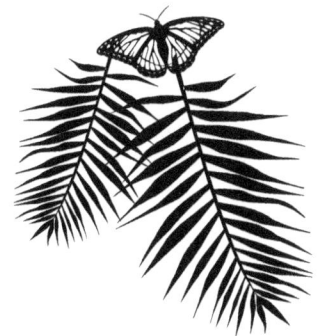

With an equatorial circumference of 24,901 miles, Planet Earth is daunting in size, yet because of improved transportation, infrastructure and technology, our massive planetary home seems to be getting smaller and smaller. Human populations are ever expanding and encroaching on pristine lands—often spontaneously creating significant environmental changes in the names of development and commercialization. Fewer and fewer places on our planet remain unexplored and undocumented by Western civilization.

Africa's Congo is a world beyond all others. Much like the realms of outer space and the deepest depths of oceans, many of its mysteries and life forms remain a secret except to those who live there.

It took almost a full year of fundraising, ten months of planning and twenty-one hours of travel for our small team of three to reach the capital city of Brazzaville, the starting point of our expedition in the Republic of the Congo.

A phone call eleven months earlier had sent my heart in a whirlwind. On the other end was a donor for Healing Seekers,

Sadie, with her spouse, Alyce, announcing the decision to fund the majority of the trek. Until that point, the Congo had been little more than a big dream.

My voice quivered in response to Sadie's words, as both shock and elation took hold. The gift was not only unsolicited but unprecedented. In fact, in years past, Healing Seekers had been unable to obtain even a tiny fraction of expedition funding from outside sources.

In the weeks that followed the phone call, generosity and kindness flowed. It was as if Sadie and Alyce's gift had opened multiple doors through which further contributions streamed. A GoFundMe campaign attracted individual donations ranging from ten dollars to thousands of dollars. With the additional donations, the remaining funds for the expedition were quickly secured.

The trek would be to one of the world's largest jungles and to an area whose flora and fauna were considered largely unknown. The specific area was also said to be one of the least explored by nonindigenous people and as such, there were but a handful of satellite images that the logistics team we had hired had been able to gather. The images were imperative in mapping our course in hopes of avoiding vast swamps, cliffs and other dead-ends.

Areas of dense vegetation were said to be so entangled with vine-like lianas, which often grew to two and three thousand feet in length, that many deemed the particular area of the jungle impenetrable. Other areas were said to have swamps that were not only tremendously difficult to navigate but were also havens for venomous snakes and crocodiles.

Because of the remote location, the trek would require a logistics team within the country and a Congolese team of porters, trackers and guides. The expedition would also become the most expensive

Chapter Twenty-Two

undertaking in Healing Seekers' history. Therefore, the number of team members leaving the U.S. was reduced from the originally anticipated six members to three.

The two members joining with me were: Eduardo, director of videography and master guide, who had been with me on every trip since the first trek in 2006. And David, a producer and filmmaker, whom I had known for forty years. It would be David's first adventure with Healing Seekers.

The positions within the team were never easy to fill. A member needed to have extensive experience in the outdoors and internationally. He or she had to be in great shape, and he or she had to be both physically and emotionally tough. The last thing anyone wanted to hear was constant complaining or whining or someone wanting to quit after the first week. Most of all, he or she had to be a team player and place the team and its mission above all else.

Eduardo and David were the perfect selections.

It was a late February afternoon when the three of us checked in at the Raleigh-Durham airport. Our route would take us from Raleigh-Durham to Atlanta to Paris to Brazzaville. The flights were smooth and provided ideal opportunities to watch movies, read and catch up on much needed sleep.

As the Paris flight began its descent into Brazzaville, I stared out the window. Through the clouds I glimpsed the land below. It was green and lush. Its canopy thick . . . just as I had imagined. Along the horizon, a flock of white birds flew into the orange-rose sky of the setting sun, almost as if their flight had been orchestrated to perfectly time with our arrival.

A few minutes later, the Congo River came into view. Its volume and magnitude were unmistakable. Formed almost two million years earlier, the river seemed to have been carved out of the jungle, winding its way through the blanket of green like a black serpent.

Although I was suspended thousands of feet above, the land below seemed to beckon me.

And its beauty took hold of my heart.

Due to our late day arrival, we would stay two nights in the capital city of Brazzaville. This would help us to adjust to the different time zone while also giving time to pack additional equipment and supplies. In Brazzaville, we would join with three members of a logistics team whom we had hired to orchestrate all the ground work, including food, supplies, porters, trackers, SUVs, boats and permits before our arrival.

The logistics team would include the owner of the logistics company, Macs, and his assistant, Bryan, both of whom resided outside the Congo but based a division of their company in the country. The third member was an indigenous Congolese guide, Nettor.

The logistics team had been hired eight months prior to the trek. A face-to-face meeting in New York with Macs set guidelines in place, while emails and phone calls over the next several months mapped out the course and planned every detail, including necessary equipment, food, supplies and medical kits.

On the morning of the third day, the six of us would leave the capital city of Brazzaville and travel north via two SUVs to the city of Ouesso, near the border with Cameroon. In Ouesso we would connect with the remaining members of our team: thirteen

Chapter Twenty-Two

trackers, porters and guides. In addition to arranging permits, transportation, food and ground supplies like generators, Macs and his team were responsible for hiring and securing the Congolese team.

Eduardo, David and I had extensively prepared for the trek. For months, we had physically trained and had rehearsed for a vast number of potential problems including medical issues, venomous snakes, back-up failures, camera problems and battery issues, especially since the life of a battery is greatly diminished with the jungle's high temperatures and humidity. Our packing was impeccable and precise, allowing only enough room for the necessities of filming, clothing and survival.

There was not one thing that was incomplete. Not one thing for which Eduardo, David and I felt unprepared.

Never had I fathomed, however, that the logistics team would neglect their duties and fall short of their responsibilities. It had only taken a few hours after our arrival to realize the logistics team's incompetency. Permits and permissions were unsecured. Food, water, equipment and supplies were both incomplete and inadequate.

As a wilderness survival expert and NOLS (National Outdoor Leadership School) instructor, Eduardo was shocked to realize that Macs, Bryan and Nettor had misled us. They were not only unprepared, they were inexperienced. The amount of food and water they had calculated was horribly deficient. When Eduardo calculated the water and food needed per person per day, it became evident that the logistics team had merely guessed at what was needed. And guessed to everyone's potential detriment.

The rations of food and water that they had secured would be depleted in five to seven days, falling terribly short of the amount needed for the weeks we would be away. Re-supply lines were impractical and inoperable with both logistics and the number of porters on hand. Far from expansive and complete, the medical kits were more suitable for an elementary school field trip. Fortunately, I had packed extensive medical kits, as I never fully trusted the medical care of my team to anyone else.

Of utmost importance to the success of the trek was a generator. Without the ability to recharge batteries and equipment and download footage, our project was dead. But instead of the two high quality generators that we had paid for and insisted upon, Macs had one cheap, marginally substandard generator that he had purchased outside of the country at a members' only warehouse company to save money. After thirty minutes of testing it, the generator stopped.

Eduardo, David and I spent most of a day searching for a dependable generator in a country where such items were rare. We walked along roads with randomly erected small shops, only feet away from the dirt streets. There were shops for clothes, tires, tools and hoses, batteries and fuel.

Most stores were smaller than twenty-by-fifty feet. They either had wide front doors that had been swung open or a single door that had been raised toward the ceiling, much like a garage door. The frontal openings allowed views of the stores' contents, which were covered in red dust that had settled from the stirrings from the dirt roads.

In the course of our search, we found two merchants who had generators, but the generators were used and looked as if they had been sitting idle for years. Finally, we came across a third merchant

Chapter Twenty-Two

who had a brand new one. Even though it had the Honda name on the box, we worried about the quality of the generator because we had been warned by a previous merchant that merchandise was often counterfeit. Some were perfectly copied while others had misspellings and were more obvious, such as the box he pointed out that was labeled Hitache instead of Hitachi.

Opening the box, we set up the generator and purchased a gallon of gas from the owner, and in the doorway of the store, the merchant started the machine. After successfully running it for almost an hour, we purchased it. And prayed that it would last the entirety of the trek.

Until our arrival in the country, Macs had portrayed himself and his team as experts in both the Congo and as logistics guides. He insisted that although they had never been to the remote region, they were more than capable of the expedition's demands. For months, the discussions with him via emails, phone calls, conference calls, and even the face-to face meeting in New York were, in hindsight, both inflated and misleading.

Correcting the logistics, supplies, equipment and calculations took enormous time and energy. Eduardo continued to teach the logistics team all the things they had pretended to know and to take the lead on all such fronts.

David took the lead on translating our English to French and vice versa. French was another skill in which Macs had claimed to be proficient but was not. David had taken three years of French in high school, twenty years earlier, and in two days spoke more fluently than Macs.

The paperwork and permits, however, which had only been filed weeks earlier and should have been completed before our arrival, remained solely in the hands of the logistics team. For us to begin the process anew would mean several additional weeks of waiting. Without the paperwork, travel to our designated region and into the jungle itself was prohibited.

    The original plan had been to overnight in Ouesso on day three. On the fourth day, we would purchase any final supplies for our team porters and trackers before traveling southeast by boat along the Sangha River to the village of Pokola. In Pokola we would spend the fourth night, departing the village the following morning for the jungle, located several hours northeast.

    But by the third day of the expedition, the well-planned itinerary we had spent months creating with Macs was both muddled and obsolete. Instead of entering the jungle on day five, we sat and waited for days in Ouesso and then in Pokola for the mandatory permits and permissions to be obtained. Each morning we awakened with anticipation of leaving for the jungle, only to be disappointed time after time with an announcement from Macs that they had not yet acquired the necessary paperwork.

    With each passing hour and each passing day, our irritation and frustration mounted. Adding to the impatience was dealing with Macs' ever-increasing negativity and fear, which included forebodings that one or more of us were going to die from malaria, venomous snakes or tribal attacks during the trek. His weakness was shocking, as he had portrayed nothing but confidence and even a cockiness in the months prior.

    Tired of the adversity and inactivity, Eduardo, David and I decided to unpack the cameras on day seven and film an introduction to our documentary at the Pokola market. The market was a half-acre of cleared land that contained rows of vendors, side-by-side. Goods were displayed either on wooden tables or on top of cloths that were spread on the ground. A simple wooden roof protected the merchants and their merchandise from the sun and rain.

Each vendor sold but a few items. Bananas, flip flops, eggs, warm Coca-Colas and woven bags were for sale, as were jeans and knit shirts of various styles and sizes. Clothing bearing the labels of Façonnable and Ralph Lauren were common and mixed in stacks with knock-off names like Nikie and Pollo.

It was not at all the introduction to our film that we had planned, but it would be interesting to show students the markets and merchandise. Plus, the filming made us feel like we were being productive.

The day was lovely, and after filming with the handheld cameras, Eduardo flew the drone over the market for an aerial perspective. We then walked through the village, stopping briefly to fly the drone over a field where two teams of young men played soccer.

Crowds gathered around us, especially the children. They loved the drone and begged us to take their pictures. Flying the drone within feet above their heads, Eduardo made the children scream with excitement as they chased after the drone, waving to it.

When daylight began to fade, we realized that the sunset over the Sangha River was destined to be spectacular, so we quickly walked through the village to the river's bank to film the last thirty minutes of daylight. As Eduardo and I stood by the river's edge flying the drone, David yelled to us from behind. Turning around, we saw David frantically walking toward us, gesturing sharply with his hand moving left to right in front of his neck as if he were slicing his neck.

"Stop! Stop the drone!" he screamed. "We're in trouble!"

Walking twenty-five feet behind David were three police officers. Following the officers were Macs, Nettor and Bryan. As they neared, the police spoke loudly in a language we did not understand and pointed to the drone, that Eduardo had only seconds earlier landed. The tone in their voices was firm and intense, yet the only words that were said in French that David understood were "you have broken the law" and "you are going to jail."

Without further translation or explanation, we were corralled toward a vehicle that had arrived only moments after the police. One by one, we were shuttled into the bed of the small white truck—Eduardo, David and myself . . . followed by Bryan, Macs and Nettor. And told to sit. And be quiet.

Standing over us and leaning against the cab of the truck was an armed guard.

The officer in charge then slammed the tailgate, looked at the guard who stood over us and nodded. He then walked toward the driver's door while the other guard walked along the right side of the truck toward the front passenger door. Getting into the truck, they slammed the doors and the head officer started the engine. And drove like a maniac.

The terrain near the river was rough. Our bodies knocked against one another as the truck slammed into crevices and holes. After finally reaching the smoother dirt of the village's main road, the officer slowed the truck considerably. As if he wanted to parade us through the village, he decelerated until the truck crept at a nominal speed, giving everyone an opportunity to stop and stare at the contents in the bed of his vehicle. Many of the villagers we passed were those we had seen only hours earlier when we were filming.

I looked at Eduardo who sat against me to my left.

Chapter Twenty-Two

Whispering, he said, "Don't worry, Amy. I can handle this."
I smiled ever so slightly. I knew he could.

The truck eventually pulled off to the side of a road and stopped. When it did, the guard in the back of the truck jumped over its side, let the tailgate down and directed us to a narrow strip of dried grass beside a long wooden fence that ran parallel to the road. Twenty feet from where we stood, the fence's solo gate was swung open by the chief officer who motioned for us to walk through.

We followed the chief officer, walking along a two-foot-wide dirt path that led from the gate to a small white and light blue building fifty feet away. When we neared its entrance, he stepped aside and directed us to enter.

Inside the building was a single large rectangular room, twelve-by-twenty feet. Five feet inside the door was a wooden desk and chair. In front of the desk, along the two side walls, were long perpendicular wooden benches that reminded me of old church pews.

And on them, we were told to sit.

Eduardo and David entered first and sat on the bench against the far wall at the end closest to the desk. I sat directly across from them, at the end of the second bench, closest to the desk and closest to the door. The logistics team filed in behind us and retreated toward the ends of the benches near the back of the room.

The walls of the room were painted multiple shades of blue, almost as if there had not been enough of one color to cover it all. Two feet above Eduardo's and David's heads was a small window. From it dangled crooked metal strips that appeared to have once been strapped tightly across the pane to prevent escape. In the ceiling above, two dim light bulbs softly lit the room. In the far back, a pile of odd wooden and metal pieces was stacked next to a fan, which slowly oscillated back and forth.

Eduardo, David and I looked at one another and whispered: "What's happening? What did we do? What's going on?"

As the questions poured, we looked at one another for some kind of reassurance that everything was going to be okay. But that didn't happen. Instead, we seemed to only reflect mirror images of shock and fear.

Looking at Macs and Nettor made matters even worse. Their nonverbal cues were pure panic. I knew at that point that although Eduardo, David and I were afraid, it would be up to us to keep the group calm, collective and rational. Panic would serve no purpose.

Moments later, the officers entered the room. The one in authority took a seat behind the desk while the other two stood like soldiers near him, only a few feet to my left, blocking the exit. The chief officer then stood and began to yell, glaring at each of us . . . one by one. Pounding his right fist on the desk, his anger escalated as the veins in his neck protruded, becoming more pronounced with each passing minute.

Our attempts to speak, to apologize or to ask for translations were met with more intense yells as if saying, "shut up."

The officer's behavior and responses evoked terror. And further confusion. Without translations, there was no understanding.

We had no voice.

We had no power.

After forty-five minutes, Nettor, who happened to be the only person capable of understanding and translating the officers' words into French, stood up with Macs and asked if they could go outside the building to talk. At their request, Eduardo, David and I stared

Chapter Twenty-Two

at one another in amazement—and mouthed the words, "What the hell? What are they doing?"

I couldn't help but think that they were about to flee, leaving us alone to bear any wrath or consequences.

Granting the request, the officer in charge then instructed one of the two guards at the door to follow and guard them.

The chief officer then turned his attention back to us and continued yelling. When he tired, the remaining officer at the door took over, more boisterous and louder than his boss.

We had no idea what they were saying, only that they were very, very angry. Every time we looked at each other and diverted our attention, they screamed even louder, often standing up and pounding on the desk as if to say, "how dare you!"

When one tired, the other resumed. And the cycle repeated itself. For almost two hours we endured the vocal lashings while attempting to understand what had happened and what was happening. Throughout the ordeal, in English and in French, we apologized and tried to explain that we intended no harm or disrespect. But before we could get out two sentences, the officers in unison spoke over us. Our interruptions only seemed to heighten their anger. No matter how hard we tried, their responses remained the same—a flurry of words we did not understand in tones of harsh reprimand and condemnation.

Finally, the head officer turned to the guard next to him and pointed to the door. The guard left and demanded that the others return. As Macs and Nettor entered, the officer in charge addressed Nettor. Nettor then turned to us and spoke. David translated his French into English.

"The chief officer told him to translate his words so that we understand fully what he is saying," David said.

As Macs and Nettor retreated once again to the back of the room, the chief officer reached into his desk drawer and pulled out a single sheet of paper. Looking up at Nettor, he spoke. As Nettor translated the officer's language to French, David continued the translations to English.

"He will now make an official arrest report," David relayed.

The chief officer looked directly at Macs and asked a series of questions. After Macs, he asked the same questions to Bryan. After Bryan, he asked Nettor, and then directed the same to me, David and Eduardo.

"What is your name? Where are you coming from? Where are you going? Why are you here? How long is your stay in the Congo? What is your occupation? What equipment do you have? What belongings do you have?"

With each response, he scribbled on the paper. At the end of questioning, he looked up and spoke for several minutes. Afterwards, Nettor sat still. The officer then raised his voice as if to force Nettor to translate.

Reluctantly, Nettor translated the words to David.

"We have been declared guilty—" David struggled to say, "and are being charged—with espionage. With spying on the village and government offices.

They are demanding the drones. Cameras. Phones. Any equipment we have used to take or record pictures in the village. Any tapes—computers. In our possession."

As David's eyes moistened, my heart sank. Slowly, he uttered the words, "We are all going to jail."

With David's translation, Eduardo spoke up and looked directly at the chief officer, "Please. Please let us show you the footage. They are photos only of children and the market and river. They are not

Chapter Twenty-Two

of government or official buildings. We are filming for education. We have permits."

David translated Eduardo's words into French and Nettor translated the French into the officer's language.

"Please," Eduardo continued, "let us show all that we have. It is for education. We are not spies."

The officer, however, didn't budge or even blink. Dismissing Eduardo's pleas, he put his head down and continued his report.

When Eduardo tried to speak again, the officer told him to be quiet. With his words, we stared at each other in silence and then watched helplessly as the officer continued to write. After a few minutes, the chief officer announced that the arrest report was complete.

He then demanded our passports.

When his words were translated, no one moved. Surrendering our passports evoked an even greater level of terror, for it loudly declared the guilty verdict. The passports were our freedom. Without them we were powerless and had no escape. Passports were required for transit through any region in the country and had been required multiple times during our travels. Without them, we could not even enter the neighboring region.

When no one moved, the officer slammed his fist forcefully on the desk and yelled.

There was no need for translation.

For a brief moment, I remained motionless and watched as Eduardo and David reached into their pockets. My thoughts swirled in a sickening spin. I turned to look at the chief officer and was startled to see that he was angrily glaring at me. Digging into the side pocket of my pants, I grabbed my passport and, with the others, handed it over.

Gathering all the passports, the head officer then stacked them in a small pile and began to meticulously go through each. One by one, he opened the passports, looking up each time to find the owner in the room. He then flipped through the pages and paused briefly before showing the page to the other two officers, pointing sternly as if the contents were condemning evidence.

After the review of the passports, the chief officer allowed us to talk.

David continued to translate our English to French while Nettor translated the French into the officer's language. We explained our work and the purpose of our filming. We showed our permit to film and explained that the filming included cameras and drones. We pleaded for the opportunity to show the footage, especially the drone footage, which was nothing more than aerial views of the market area, two teams playing soccer on a grassy field and beauty shots of the river.

At first, the chief officer declined. But we persisted to the point that Eduardo boldly stood and began to unpack the computer and eject the memory cards from the cameras before placing the laptop on the edge of the officer's desk. Although hesitant, the chief officer finally agreed to watch the footage.

The three men hovered behind Eduardo, leaning over his shoulders to stare at the computer's screen. After a few minutes, they leaned in further, pointing and laughing.

After seeing the footage, the chief and the two subordinate officers stepped outside. Fifteen minutes later they returned, and he explained that we would be released upon a monetary payment.

At the announcement, Macs spoke up for the first time. He proudly explained that he and Nettor had gone outside earlier to offer a monetary payment. Unbeknownst to us, Macs and Nettor had bribed the officer who was guarding them, who then took the offer to the chief officer.

Chapter Twenty-Two

With the payment, we would be released and our passports returned.

Grateful for our release, we thanked the chief officer and followed his two subordinates out of the building, down the dirt path and through the gate. We piled into the back of the same white truck, this time driven by the officer who had been persuaded to take the bribe, and made our way back to the guesthouse where we were staying. While Eduardo, David and I went inside and gathered the money, the driver waited with the members of the logistics team by the vehicle.

The money was pulled from our cash reserve, which was to be used in the case of an emergency. Thank God we had prepared.

The 500,000 CFA francs was the equivalent to almost nine hundred U.S. dollars. It was a considerable amount of money in the Congo, almost twice the country's average annual household income.

I walked to the vehicle and gave the stack of money to Macs, who then handed it to the officer with whom he had negotiated the bribe. Moments later, the officer drove away.

Macs, however, did not have the passports even though it was part of the deal. Instead, he stated that the passports were going to be returned the following morning after being stamped by an immigration official.

"What immigration official? What stamp? Are our passports being flagged? Are they documenting the arrest in our passports?" Eduardo, David and I asked.

"Are you sure we are going to get them back?" I asked.

"You should never have given the money until the passports were returned," argued Eduardo, while David chimed, "Man, that was not smart. What if we have to pay more money? What if we don't get them back?"

Macs looked confused, but provided no answers and instead, walked away.

Worrying that our passports would not be returned without further issue led to a long and restless night. I feared that our troubles were not over.

It was seven o'clock the next morning when Eduardo, David and I made our way through the village to a gathering place for coffee and eggs. The building was simple and clean, with five wooden tables inside and two wooden picnic tables outside. A young man utilized a small grill and an oven to offer a breakfast menu of eggs, fruit and bread.

Behind the small kitchen area, a covered walkway led to a larger wooden building with several rooms, which were primarily rented by executives and employees of the local logging company when they were in the village.

The plan that morning was for the logistics team to meet us at eight o'clock for breakfast. But as was the norm, the logistics team failed to show up on time. Or even within the hour.

Several hours later, Macs, Nettor and Bryan graced us with their presence.

As Macs sat, he began to reprimand and chastise us for the arrest . . . for filming with the drone in the village and even condemning Eduardo for taking photos with his cell phone.

"Your actions have caused a lot of problems," he fumed. "The arrest was very serious. We could have gone to jail for months. Maybe forever. We could have died here. You have caused a lot of trouble.

The village, the chief and the elders are all upset with you."

Chapter Twenty-Two

After a brief pause, he continued, "We are being asked to leave. We will most likely be permanently banned from the country.

The trek is over. Here are your passports.

I have arranged a vehicle, that will arrive for you tomorrow morning at nine o'clock to transport you back to Brazzaville. From there, you will go back to the United States."

Macs' words were incomprehensible. It was as if I was having a nightmare from which I could not awaken. First, it was absurd that they were calling off the expedition. The problem and the arrest had been resolved, and as soon as they secured the permits, we would be leaving the village and going to the jungle.

Second, it was unfathomable that we had done something so wrong that it had upset the village to the point that we were being asked to leave. The village had been friendly since the very first day, smiling and waving to us as we walked through the village multiple times a day. There had to be a misunderstanding—and for that, we needed to apologize, discuss and correct.

Finally, I could not begin to imagine how I would explain the failure to Sadie and Alyce and our many supporters back home. Much less, admit that we had been asked to leave a country, even before entering the jungle.

After the meeting, Eduardo, David and I walked slowly through the village back to the guesthouse. The sadness was overwhelming. It was as if we had committed some unpardonable sin. And yet, something just wasn't right. Although we talked nonstop, I cannot recall the conversation. Only that each of us became so emotional, we struggled hard to fight back the tears.

Although I was angry, Eduardo and David were furious. Like me, they expressed their distrust with the logistics team, wondering if this was all staged to end a trek for which they were obviously ill-prepared and unqualified.

At the guesthouse, I went directly to the right corner of my room and sat on the floor. It was the furthest point from the door and also the corner where my soft North Face dry bags were piled. Lying across them, I cupped my hands to my face and quietly and mournfully sobbed. Softly, I cried out in angst and in anger . . .

At God.

With fury, I demanded to know why the trek was being canceled. Why had we not been spared the problems? Why had our path not been cleared of obstacles? What had I done to deserve this? What had I done to warrant such punishment for the team and the organization?

The canceled trek would likely lead to the demise of Healing Seekers. No one would support a project that could not guarantee some measurable outcome, like the educational materials we had always provided from an expedition.

Until our arrival in the country, everything with the trek had been flawless—beginning with Sadie and Alyce's gift, then the fundraising, preparations and planning. But when the logistics team entered the picture, it seemed every door that had once been opened was slammed shut. One thing after another had bedeviled the trip: extensive delays that compromised the trek's full itinerary and purpose, additional expenses of lodging while waiting on permits - transportation, food, equipment and supplies that had to be recalculated and rearranged. And finally, the arrest and its financial hit . . . followed by the devastating cancellation of the trek.

My conversation with God was severe and intense. I crossed lines I had never dared. Anger, sadness and frustration cycled until the tears and grieving gave way to emotional exhaustion. Curling up into the fetal position, I closed my eyes and released a long, slow sigh.

Chapter Twenty-Two

An hour later, a gentle knock at my door shook me from my stupor. Wiping my face, I got up to find Eduardo and David at the door insisting that we not give up. Something, they claimed, did not make sense. Something wasn't right.

Since our arrival, the locals had been friendly and kind. In Pokola especially, groups had gravitated toward us and we, toward them. And they had loved the drone and the footage. We had made many friends, unlike Macs and Nettor, who rarely even acknowledged anyone they passed.

If we had offended anyone, why had the responses from the community members not reflected it? We therefore began to seek out our Pokola friends and ask them directly. If we had upset them and were being forced to leave, we would NOT leave without apologizing.

To our surprise, every person with whom we spoke insisted that we had done nothing wrong and had upset no one. We then went to the chief of the village and she, likewise, stated that we had done nothing to upset anyone. She continued by saying that she had heard of the arrest and apologized for the way that we had been treated. She thanked us for coming to see her, for it was something that the logistics team had not done.

After speaking to several people in the village and to the village chief, Eduardo, David and I sought the advice of the person we trusted most and the one on whom we knew we could depend.

It would take almost two hours to travel by vehicle on a back road to reach an area where we could pay for a boat to transport us across the river to the city of Ouesso. Ouesso was where we could find our friend, Denise. It was during the days that we had waited in Ouesso for the logistics team to acquire the appropriate permits that

And the Silent Spoke

we spent hours with her each day at the restaurant she owned. She was also one of the very few people in the area who spoke English.

Denise was a beautiful woman with striking green eyes and gorgeous dark brown, shoulder-length hair. Her mother was Congolese and her father, French. She was like an angel who watched over us each day, protecting us while expressing her frustration at the way we were being treated and not cared for by the company we had hired. Denise had become more than a friend and trusted adviser; she had become our Congolese mother.

Returning to the restaurant, we sat and recounted the arrest and the decision by the logistics team to end the trek. As we shared the story, Denise became very upset.

"Lies. Lies. Lies," she exclaimed. "This company who claims to be of the Congo is not Congo. They are bad people. You have done nothing wrong. It is not wrong to film.

The elders would never be angry over such things. These are lies."

Taking a deep breath, she continued, "We will help you. Please stay. It is important for people to see how good and beautiful our country is. This is not Congo . . . they are not Congo.

Please don't leave."

With her encouragement and her insistence, we agreed to stay.

As we sat with Denise, a phone call came through on the satellite phone from Macs, who had no idea that we had traveled back to Ouesso. I announced the decision that the three of us were continuing the trek without him and that he should cancel the vehicle he had arranged to pick us up the following morning.

Angrily he stipulated that we had no right to stay and had no choice but to leave. But I responded that since it was he who had called off the trek, we were no longer officially affiliated. And with my words, he ended the call.

Chapter Twenty-Two

Ten minutes later, however, another call came through from an unknown number. On the other end was a man who introduced himself as Macs' business partner who was based in the neighboring country of the Democratic Republic of the Congo, in the capital city of Kinshasa.

With a voice that was irate and commanding, he spoke nonstop. Yelling into the phone, he demanded that we leave the country immediately while claiming to have friends nearby within the local military forces who would, at his request, arrest and take us away. Never to be seen again.

"We are not affiliated with Macs any longer." I rebutted. "We are continuing without them. In fact, we don't want anything to do with them anymore. They will go their way and we will go ours."

He nonetheless continued his tirade, threatening to have his friends locate us within the hour, hurt us and take us away if we failed to follow Macs' instructions.

With his final threat of inflicting harm upon us and taking us away, I told him I would call off the trek. Such an imprisonment could place our families and friends in extremely difficult situations, from dealing with our sudden disappearance to the possible payment of ransoms for our release . . . not to mention the possible physical and emotional harm. This, I could not justify.

The phone call was the final blow. We could not compete against such corruption. We could not take such a risk.

Shaken, I hung up the phone and relayed the conversation to Eduardo, David and Denise.

Eduardo and David sat in shock while Denise excused herself and walked several feet away to make two calls with her cell phone. Shortly thereafter, both the Congolese Ambassador to Russia and a highly respected businessman in Ouesso who had connections to high-ranking military officers in the country were sitting at our table.

Both men were outraged with the story, especially with the logistics team's tactics and corrupt behavior. They were embarrassed that we had been led to pay a bribe, as bribes were illegal in the country. But most of all, they were livid at the logistics team's threat of imprisonment.

It was the very opposite image they wished outsiders to have of their country.

Within an hour of the Ambassador's arrival, our story and situation escalated to Denis Sassou Nguesso, the President of the Republic of the Congo. The President immediately ordered an investigation to be led by a colonel who presided over all the region and its law enforcement bodies. With the Presidential decree, the Colonel demanded a meeting the following morning in his office in Ouesso to review the circumstances. Those required to attend the meeting were the three members of the logistics team, the officers who had arrested us, and representatives of our team.

Representing our team would be David, our French-speaking teammate who had been proven to have excellent communication skills especially in conflict situations, and Joseph, the local businessman who understood the regional laws and regulations and who also spoke both the local dialect and French.

The meeting was a great relief, for it would be an opportunity to finally understand what had happened and why we had been asked to leave. With the announcement of the meeting, Eduardo, David and I left Ouesso and made the journey back to Pokola for the night.

When we arrived at the guesthouse in Pokola, we were told by the caretaker, Donileon, that two military helicopters had landed

Chapter Twenty-Two

only an hour earlier on the outskirts of the village, close to the gathering place where we had coffee and eggs each morning. The two military pilots had arrived unannounced and were said to be staying in two of the rooms in the building behind the kitchen area.

No one in the community, we were told, ever recalled seeing such aircraft in the village.

No one knew why they had arrived.

No one knew why they stayed.

It was early the next morning when we began the journey back to Ouesso to Denise's restaurant. After a quick cup of coffee, David left with Joseph to walk the several blocks to the Colonel's office for the mandatory meeting to speak on our behalf. Eduardo and I remained at the restaurant.

What we had anticipated would be an hour-long meeting turned into half a day. Eduardo and I worried about David and contemplated going to the Colonel's office to be with him, but we worried that our appearance would be intrusive and might deter from David's authority as the spokesman for our group.

Although I worried, I knew David could handle anything that came up. If he needed us, he would have sent word through Joseph.

David had been eager to confront the logistics team. He was outraged over the lies, deception and manipulation in which we had been entrapped, and he was relentless in fighting until truth prevailed. Even if that meant we had also done something wrong.

No matter the outcome, it would only be in such strength that darkness was brought to light. And the wrong made right.

The meeting was long.

According to David, the office was cramped, hot and stuffy.

"We were all packed into this tiny space," he said. "Chairs were brought in and placed in front of the Colonel's desk. Everyone was there: Macs, Nettor and Bryan, the three arresting officers, Joseph and me. Everyone was so uptight and anxious.

Well—except for Joseph and me. We were the only ones eager for the meeting.

Macs was nervous as hell. Sweat was dripping down his face and he kept leaning over, whispering to Nettor. It was unreal how nervous he was.

In the beginning of the meeting, the Colonel asked each person in the room to tell about the arrest. One by one, each of us told pretty much the same story. When it was my turn, I gave a lot more details than the others, including how we had been left alone without a translator during the interrogation while Macs and Nettor went outside the building for more than thirty minutes, which we found out later was to negotiate the bribe. And how we didn't know anything that was going on until we were told by Macs and Nettor that everything would be okay if we just paid the money.

When it was Macs' turn, he stuttered and spoke so softly the Colonel got irritated and had to keep telling him to speak up. He ended up only giving the broadest of details.

After everyone told their own version of the story, the Colonel asked to see our film permit, which I handed over. No one said a word while he read it. Then, he stood up and with this stern tone, read out loud every word of the permit.

Chapter Twenty-Two

When he finished reading, he slammed the piece of paper on the desk and asked the officers how it could possibly have been misinterpreted. He stared at the officers, but not one of them spoke. The officers wouldn't even look up at him.

The Colonel then looked at me and said not to worry and not to be afraid. That we had done nothing wrong.

'What was wrong,' he said, 'was negotiating and paying a bribe.'

Now this is where he gets really angry," David recounted.

"He raised his voice and pointed to each of the three officers and then to Macs, Bryan and Nettor, and said, 'You know better. You know these actions are illegal!'

He was infuriated with Macs and Nettor, saying that they were at fault for initiating and negotiating the bribe. He berated them and then banned them from ever doing business in this part of the country again! Then he forbade Nettor from ever entering this region of the country again!"

David took a deep breath and continued, "Macs was freaking out. And so was Nettor. They were terrified they were going to jail.

When the Colonel finished, Joseph asked the Colonel's help in making Macs turn over all equipment, food and supplies before they left the region, which we had paid in full and which were needed for the expedition. The Colonel then turned to Macs and Nettor and demanded them to do so.

I interjected to make sure the equipment included the satellite phone, permits, maps, images, flashlights, headlamps and batteries."

David smiled, "Then the Colonel declared that he was creating a document that would serve as a record of the facts, citing his verdict that the officers and logistics team were at fault and that we had done nothing wrong.

It took two hours just to draft the paper! I couldn't understand what was taking so long, but I didn't care. I really liked the Colonel and I respected that he was being so thorough.

After the document was written, the Colonel said that everyone would sign it. When it was Macs' turn to sign, he was sweating and his face was beet red.

The Colonel said copies would be made and the original would be sent to President Denis Sassou Nguesso.

The Colonel then looked at me and said that the President was very upset over the situation and at the way we had been treated and that the President is demanding that the money be returned.

I suggested the money be given to the community, but the Colonel said that we had to take all of it back.

Then, he said that the President wants the world to know that the people of the Congo are good people and that acts such as these are unacceptable."

Looking at Eduardo and then at me, David went on to say, "The President wants us to continue our journey. And you're not going to believe this—he said that our situation has encouraged him to make available more opportunities for organizations like ours to come to the Congo.

And he wishes us well.

Can you believe that?"

My respect for David had never been greater. He handled the situation impeccably, holding tight to the highest of moral standards. He protected and defended not only us, but the Congolese people, such as our porters and trackers who also had been mistreated by the logistics team and who had not been given a voice.

Chapter Twenty-Two

Two hours after the meeting's end, David, Eduardo and I met with Macs and Nettor to collect the supplies and equipment. After we checked off all the items on our list, the logistics team frantically loaded their personal bags into an SUV and fled.

With their departure, a refreshing empowerment took hold.

Eduardo, David and I returned to the restaurant and sat with Denise and Joseph. And toasted with cold beer. Shortly thereafter, a police official arrived and handed us an envelope. Stuffed inside was 500,000 CFA francs.

I thought about the days leading up to the meeting with the Colonel and couldn't help but to think that there was a higher purpose for the logistics team's departure. For I believe that had they continued with us, the purity and sacredness of the mission and the expedition itself would have been compromised. And tainted.

And so, it was with their exodus that we eagerly began our journey anew.

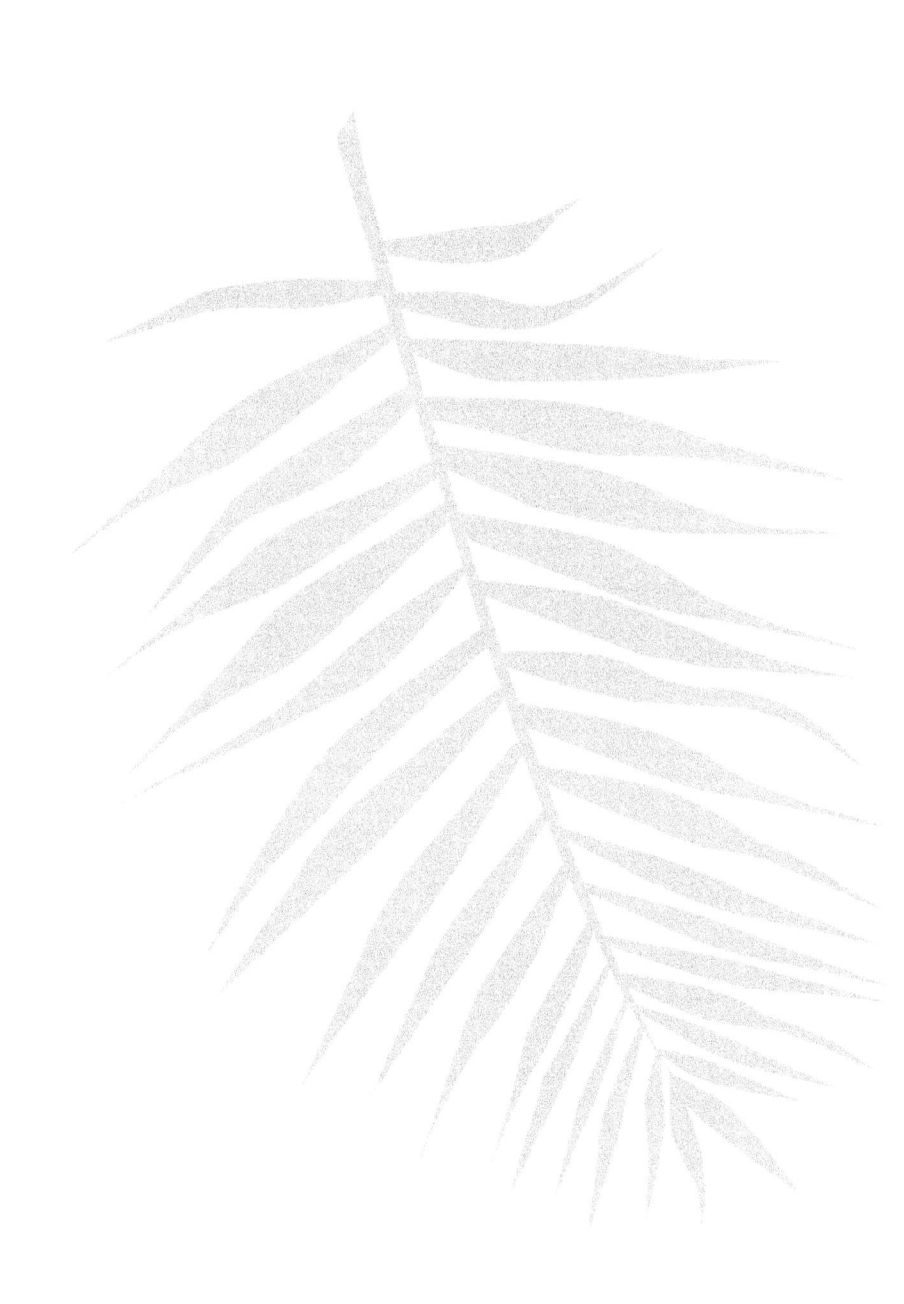

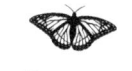

Chapter Twenty-Three

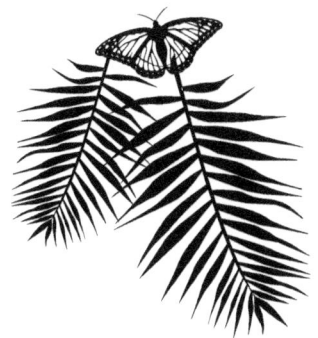

Over the next two days, we continued to learn of things left undone by the logistics company. Porters, trackers and guides, for example, had been waiting like us for days in Ouesso and then in Pokola at the request of Macs, the leader of the logistics team. They, however, had not been given any pay or compensation, water or food during the days they waited. Even though we had paid for that and more.

The departure of the three-member logistics team considerably reduced the supplies, food and necessities we would need to haul during the trek. However, it also meant that we would not need all the porters, especially the ones who had been hired to carry the logistics team's supplies and provisions. Letting go of several porters was very difficult, as each man had faithfully waited each day under Macs's instruction, eager to participate in the journey.

If we could have kept every man, we would have. But our finances prevented it. Macs had fled without reimbursing any of the money we had paid him, stating that he had no money left. Not only had we paid in full for his services, we had also paid him in full for the provisions and the services of every porter, tracker and guide for the entire trek.

Refusing to call off the trek due to the lack of money, I made several calls with the satellite phone back to the U.S. and arranged for money to be wired through Western Union with the help of my partner and our Healing Seekers' bookkeeper, Theresa. Within twenty-four hours, the funds arrived in Pokola.

During those days, we helped correct the wrongs, obtain the necessary permits and permissions, locate reliable drivers and vehicles and plan additional possible medical emergencies with the local medical clinic. We worked quickly and efficiently with the porters, trackers and guides, making sure they had all the provisions and supplies they needed and were given all that they had been promised. Together, we made a strong and solid team.

To manage the team of porters and trackers was our head guide, Donald, who quickly decided which members of the original team would continue with us and which ones would not. Handsome and intelligent, and at six-feet-two-inches-tall, Donald presented as a man of great strength and authority. Yet, when he spoke, he did so with a gentleness that made everyone listen attentively.

Charting the course within the jungle would be the job of our head tracker, Matoo, who was known as one of the best trackers in the area. He was quiet, shy and rarely made eye contact, appearing deep in thought one minute and giggling like a child the next. Deep crescent-shaped facial lines ran from either side of his nose to the corners of his mouth, while several scars marked other parts of his face, including a round one-inch spot on his upper right cheek

Chapter Twenty-Three

close to his eye, perhaps the result of a severe burn. As a member of the Baka tribe (or Bayaka, as they are known in the Congo), he was also referred to and known by the generic term, pygmy—a word that was commonly used by Macs, but often considered derogatory.

The Baka people's smaller stature, which was typically no more than four-feet-eleven-inches, had intrigued researchers in other parts of the world for many years. Some thought the shorter height was the result of deficiencies in calcium or possibly vitamin D, while others speculated there could be issues with a growth hormone. I wondered, however, if the height was instead a dominant trait. One which helped them to better navigate the dense jungle and helped to ensure their survival.

While Donald would serve as the head guide and Matoo as the head tracker, the remaining members of the team would serve as porters. Strong and physically fit, they would carry the heavier packs filled with food, supplies, equipment and gear. Two of them, known for their skills with tracking, would also assist Matoo.

To reach our targeted section of the jungle, we would need to travel two of the roads operated by the local logging company. The day prior to our scouting trip, in which we would determine our exact point of entry into the jungle, we visited the logging company to ask permission to travel their roads, even though Donald said it was not necessary.

With the permission of several officials with the logging company, we gathered early the following morning, piled into the open bed of a Toyota truck driven by a man who lived in the village. Departed Pokola and headed north to scout the area.

And the Silent Spoke

The logging road, barely wide enough for the company's eighteen wheelers with their hauls of only one, two or three of the jungle's gigantic trees, was enveloped on either side by dense foliage. Three times, spotting the enormous loads coming down the road in our direction, our driver pulled off the side of the road into the foliage to allow room for the eighteen-wheeler to pass. In the large truck's wake, tall plumes of red dirt swirled into the air, blanketing our bodies with layers of dry, dusty particles.

"The roads took much time to make," Donald announced and David translated. "The logging company works closely with the villages here. Everyone likes them.

Someone from the logging company goes into the forest with one or two members of the village to decide which trees will be cut. They mark the trees, so that when they come back, they know which ones to cut down.

They will only cut down one tree in an area and leave the other trees alone. This way the forest isn't hurt. It can recover quickly and keep growing.

The logging company employs many people. They provide jobs, housing, health care and schools. Children are educated. Everyone is happy."

After hours of driving, we veered off the first logging road onto a second, less traveled one, which formed the southern border of the swath of forest we would explore. When we reached the area we had charted for our entry into the jungle, the driver stopped the vehicle and we all got out.

Slowly, Matoo walked ahead of everyone else along the left side

Chapter Twenty-Three

of the road, searching for a natural opening or an animal trail that would serve as an easy entry. But the outer band of grassy vegetation, which rose four to five feet in height, and the layers upon layers of plants, trees and vines beyond it made such a find difficult.

Four times, we slashed through the growth to create the beginnings of a path, only to discover an impasse such as a deep ravine or vast networks of thick vines that would have taken hours to cut through. Decisions for not pursuing a path were also based on the fact that the porters would be toting seventy- to eighty-pound packs while Donald, Matoo, Eduardo, David and I would be carrying forty-five-to fifty-pound packs. Slashing through thick areas with machetes would not only take considerable time but would also expend a great deal of energy. Going down a ravine was not bad, but having to climb up the other side, pulling yourself up by roots and trees, would be physically exhausting with the additional pack weight.

In time, we found a viable entry point. Even though signal reception was sporadic, Eduardo marked nearby coordinates with the GPS while two porters marked the spot with a small fallen tree. We then loaded back into the vehicle and drove the several hours back to Pokola.

The next morning, we awakened before sunrise. To our surprise, the caretaker of the guesthouse, Donileon, had gotten up even earlier and made coffee and eggs. Donileon had been a blessing, and it was in the many days waiting on the logistics team and during and after the arrest that she had also encouraged us to continue our trek. She assisted greatly with finding reliable drivers, securing last

And the Silent Spoke

minute food supplies and arranging transportation. As we hugged good-bye, she teared.

"I will pray for you," she said as Donald translated her language into French and David translated the French into English. "Where you are going is very dangerous. I pray to God to keep you safe and healthy. I will be here when you return."

With bags packed and with gear piled high, our team of ten boarded the two vehicles driven by Donileon's friends, left the village of Pokola and headed toward our entry point along the jungle's southern edge.

Later, Donileon would tell us that we were not the only ones to leave Pokola that morning.

Only hours after we departed, so did the military helicopters.

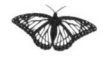
Chapter Twenty-Four

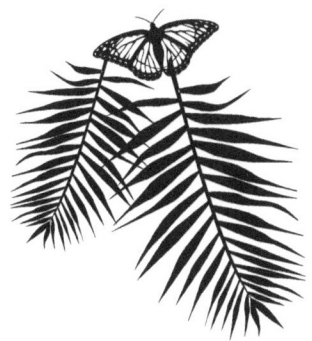

Nearing the GPS coordinates that Eduardo had documented, the drivers of both vehicles slowed to a stop. The fallen tree that had been used to mark the path we had made only hours earlier, however, was no longer visible. It was as if the jungle's flora, with its tall, thick, grassy brush, had swallowed it up overnight.

Matoo, Donald and the two porters who were also trackers walked along the side of the road searching for the fallen tree and the partially slashed path beyond it. But could not find it. Matoo stepped into the foliage and quickly disappeared. Ten minutes later, he whistled.

Much like the call of a bird, the whistle had two short, high-pitched notes followed by a third, longer one. As he continued to whistle, he emerged from the brush and pointed toward the woods. And then walking several feet in the direction of the vehicles, he pointed to the ground, where the tree lay hidden.

With the entry point located, we unloaded the gear and went over the trek's plan a final time with the two drivers. We would be gone for four weeks, maybe longer depending on what we discovered and what we confronted. Regardless, they were to keep their phones nearby at all times. If there was an emergency, we would need them to return quickly. When we phoned, we would give them directions to our location based on the entry point, which we were marking again with two fallen trees pulled next to the road.

If we came out of the jungle's northern, southern or western borders, we would eventually cross a logging road. But if we went east and then walked south along the west bank of the Ubangi River, we would eventually encounter the mighty Congo River at a point south of Mbandaka, a city located along the Congo River in the neighboring Democratic Republic of the Congo.

The Congo's waters were dangerous and deadly. Trying to navigate the powerful river or a land path beside it would be treacherous.

"He says we should stay far away from the river." David translated as Donald spoke. "The river will quickly capsize a boat. One or more of us will likely die."

"His greatest fear," David continued, "is not the river, but the possible encounters with other tribes. It sounds like he's saying militia groups . . . or armed groups. Especially those from across the river in the Democratic Republic."

With Donald's warning, we reiterated to Matoo and the trackers the original plan to go northwest and to stay away from the east.

With Matoo leading, we followed in a single line and entered the jungle's embrace.

At four-feet-three-inches-tall, Matoo was known to move swiftly and with ease within the forests. But in this region, his size and agility had little advantage. The jungle was like a never-ending matrix of growth composed of a complicated network of vines, plants and trees. Thorny briers were ubiquitous and sliced through

Chapter Twenty-Four

hands, legs, arms and torsos like sharp razor blades.

Even with ten machetes slashing through the dense foliage, our team barely altered the scene. So thick was the vegetation that if you lingered even fifteen to twenty feet behind the person ahead, it became difficult to locate the path that had just been cut.

"David, are you okay?" I would call when I turned around to find him missing.

"Where are you, Amy?" he would answer.

"Follow my voice, I'm right here."

"Guys," Eduardo, who walked ahead of me would say. "Guys, where are you?"

Although we were not far away from one another, the thick growth greatly inhibited our view. We most often became separated from one another due to the need to stop and disengage from the thorny vines that tangled with our packs, clothing and skin. To minimize damage and pain, the barbs had to be pulled away gently and carefully, and it was in those few moments that the ones in front further separated themselves from the one entangled.

Because of the jungle's thickness, progress was slow. Stops were frequent and sudden. Even though the stops allowed brief moments to stand still and rest, they also gave opportunities for the jungle to make its presence known in other ways.

Ants seemed to appear from nowhere and multiplied by the minute. They crawled over our boots, up our legs and torsos. They scurried across the leaves and branches that pressed against our bodies, making their way up our arms, backs and necks. Some were tiny . . . some were large . . . some had mandibles and bit . . . some did not. The ones that bit were painful, and often even after they were dead, the only way to rid ourselves of them was to pull their bodies away from our flesh.

After five hours of hacking through the growth, the jungle's denseness began to thin. As if we were emerging from a long dark hole, the jungle opened up and became brighter. We could finally see the extent of the tree canopy above—its matrix so thick that it blocked the sun's rays from reaching the forest floor.

Hardwoods like teak, giant fig trees, ebony and moabi were massive. With diameters of five, seven, ten feet and more, and upwards of one hundred and fifty and two hundred feet in height, the trees dominated the area. The trees in the Congo, thought to be much larger in stature than those in the Amazon, were vital producers of oxygen. They also contained great amounts of carbon due to their absorption of carbon dioxide.

With the jungle's clearing, we took off our packs and sat for the first time. One of the porters inhaled deeply and exhaled loudly, smiled and spoke in his native language. Donald translated his words into French and David translated them into English.

"He said for us to breathe," David remarked. "That this is new air. Air that no man has ever breathed before."

I closed my eyes and for a few moments, just breathed. But then, a flying insect flittered close to my face. Opening my eyes, a white butterfly with black dots along the edges of its wings landed on my left sleeve, close to my wrist. Another soon appeared and landed on my shoulder followed by two more, landing on my arms. They were majestic and elegant, painted by the most supreme artist.

The sleeves upon which they rested, however, like every thread of clothing on my body, was filthy. Saturated in sweat, it clung tightly to my skin.

Only days earlier, the shirt had been a clean, light yellow expedition shirt. Now, it was more yellowish-brown and blotched with numerous dark spots and streaks. The darkened areas were not

Chapter Twenty-Four

from dirt, but from the thorns and briers that had punctured and slashed my flesh, leaving behind smudges and trails of blood.

I looked at my teammates . . . and saw the same. David's rolled up sleeves exposed no less than thirty scratches and gashes on his forearms and hands. Above his right eye and across his face was a line of dried blood, which came from an encounter with a vine of sharp thorns that had embedded into his jaw, across his cheek, eyelid and into his scalp.

Squatting beside me, Donald held out a small one-ounce bottle. Turning it upside down, he poured a few drops of its oily mixture onto his index finger and then spread the contents over several small gashes on my face and arms. And then did likewise for each member of the team before treating himself.

The butterflies appeared in greater numbers, often landing briefly as if to say "hello" before flying off. I listened as their wings flapped near my ears, making sounds much like that of hummingbirds.

Their whisperings, however, were soon replaced with the buzzing of bees.

One, two.

Ten, twenty, forty.

The bees surrounded each of us, landing on our hands, backs, arms and legs. I stood up and looked for a hive, which I felt sure was close by. But I didn't see one. Fearing that someone might be allergic or that one or more of us might get multiple stings and have an allergic reaction, I quickly walked over to my pack, unzipped the top pocket and grabbed two EpiPens and several tablets of Benadryl. Before placing them in the side pockets of my pants, I held them up and called out to Eduardo and David. Seeing the pens, they opened the top pockets of their backpacks and each grabbed an EpiPen.

One by one, Eduardo, David and I showed each other in which shirt or pants pocket the life-saving medications were going to be stored. I then gave each of them several tablets of Benadryl to keep in the same locations.

Matoo motioned for us to move and we quickly obliged. With a pace much faster than usual, he led us slightly off-course to a route that allowed a faster escape. The heightened clip caused us to breathe much harder and sweat more profusely, but the further away we trekked, the fewer the bees. Until there were none.

Every time we stopped to rest, however, the bees reappeared. The longer we sat, the greater their numbers. Constantly on my mind was the ever-increasing possibility of someone having an anaphylactic reaction. With hundreds of bees, possibly thousands, and with only four EpiPens for our team of ten, my anxiety heightened.

What would happen if multiple members of the team faced life-threatening reactions at the same time? How would I, or any of us, make such a decision on who would receive the life-saving injections . . . and who would not?

The bees not only made it impossible to rest for a period of time, but also to film the educational materials without injury. By the time the cameras and audio were unpacked and prepped, the bees were already in vast numbers. Nonetheless, Eduardo held still the camera and David held sturdy the boom even as they quietly moaned with each sting.

I stood next to them as they refused to flinch even though the insects swarmed. Bees crawled all over Eduardo's hands, up his neck and on his face while David parted the limbs of a nearby tree

Chapter Twenty-Four

in order to raise the audio boom, only to discover that when he bent his arms, he trapped several bees who simultaneously stung the areas between his biceps and forearms. Yet, he never lowered the boom. And Eduardo never put down the camera.

Colobus monkeys jumped from limb to limb as we darted beneath them along the forest floor. Openings in the canopy made by fallen trees permitted the best opportunities to film them, as well as one particular male gorilla who seemed intrigued with our presence.

Directly above us, the western lowland gorilla straddled the trunk of a tree and stared below. Beating his chest, he leaned further toward us, as if to get a better look before beating his chest once more. Moments later, he pounded the sides of the tree multiple times before eventually urinating in our direction. Not wanting to upset him and also needing to get away from the large swarm of bees that had surrounded us, we turned off the cameras and walked away.

Our only refuge from the bees was to briskly walk away, placing greater and greater distance between us and them. But there were times when walking away was not an option.

In the early afternoons, our porters and trackers would ask to stop so that they could build a fire and prepare food. Eduardo, David and I opted for quick and easy lunches of power bars, dried fruit and trail mix. Although we offered all of our food to our teammates, they preferred a hearty cooked meal. So each day, we stopped so that a small space could be cleared and a fire started.

In a battered black pot, one of the men placed a small amount of water and heated it. From a fly-covered plastic bag, he then took several pieces of dried fish and placed them in the boiling water.

In another pot, ground yucca was mixed with water. The mixture, called *fufu*, looked like a gooey ball of dough. After kneading the dough for several minutes with a wooden stick, the bundle was pulled apart into smaller segments. Each man received a piece of fish and a portion of the fufu, which he dipped into the juice of the fish and ate.

The afternoon stops were tough. Eduardo, David and I waited patiently as the porters and trackers cooked and ate. The bees in the meantime continued to arrive in ever-higher numbers, to the point where I would often count twenty to thirty bees on the front of just one leg.

Even though walking away helped to lessen their numbers, venturing into the surrounding woods without indigenous eyes meant a greater likelihood of encounters with deadly snakes and other creatures. Even with a machete, the odds that Eduardo, David and I would respond first to something like a Gaboon viper were not good.

I looked intently for green and black mambas, pit vipers and the like, yet it was almost impossible to differentiate the vines and twigs from serpents. Making matters worse was the impaired vision I had with glasses that were constantly streaked with sweat and splotched with dirt.

I knew the snakes were out there, somewhere. In fact, it had been during the fourth day in the jungle that Matoo suddenly stopped and held up his hand for everyone to halt. Turning to his right, he pointed to a spot on the ground five feet away before turning his head slightly and speaking quietly to Donald, who stood two feet behind him.

"Serpent," Donald translated.

Matoo turned around further and motioned for us to slowly

Chapter Twenty-Four

come forward. While I quietly walked around Donald's left side, Eduardo silently took off his backpack and grabbed his second camera. Standing inches behind Matoo, I looked at the ground but could not see the snake. Matoo then leaned forward and pointed again, but I still failed to see the creature.

Behind me, Donald took a step closer, and with his motion, the viper moved.

A Gaboon viper.

With varying patterns and hues of brown, beige and black, the snake's body and triangular head were perfectly camouflaged against the forest floor. Its head looked like a dead leaf, making it almost impossible to differentiate the serpent from the natural debris.

With fangs that may reach two inches or more in length, the Gaboon viper was believed to have one of the highest venom yields of any snake. In the world. Its head was massive compared to its neck, and the length of its body, elusive.

By the time Eduardo and David were able to get closer with the cameras, the viper turned away from us and slowly slithered away.

The bees, on the other hand, were far from concealment.

We had no idea where they were coming from but assumed the swarms we encountered multiple times a day were coming from different hives. Unfortunately, nothing appeared to deter them. Facial netting, DEET, citronella . . . not even the campfires, as the bees seemed to delight in both the smoke and heat.

Swarms engulfed us day after day, during rest breaks and while waiting on our teammates to eat, and it became almost unbearable.

And the Silent Spoke

The bees appeared to be drawn to moisture and the sweat from our bodies. Unfortunately, I sweated profusely, and my completely saturated body attracted no less than a couple hundred bees.

Although the bees didn't sting immediately, they would inadvertently become trapped in our clothing, wedged in the bends of our arms and legs or sandwiched between our backs and packs—and sting. I could handle the temporary discomfort and pain of the stings, but where I struggled was with the psychological challenge of having hundreds of insects simultaneously crawling all over my body, including in my ears and between my glasses and eyes.

Eduardo, David and I vacillated between staying close to the porters and trackers where they cooked, to venturing off into the woods where we walked in sporadic patterns within a circumference of forty to fifty feet. But no matter what we did, there was no reprieve from the bees. They were everywhere. Small swarms seemed to follow each of us, just like the cloud of dirt that trailed the Peanuts character, Pig-Pen.

For whatever reason, on one particular day and at one particular hour, I hit a breaking point.

With eyes tearing up, I looked to Eduardo and David and said, "I don't know how much more I can handle."

Eduardo immediately turned, walked over to his backpack and returned with his only remaining dry pair of pants, insisting that I put them on.

"Put these on, Amy. They will avert the onslaught," he said.

"No, Eduardo. Thank you, but I am not taking your last pair of dry pants," I responded.

"Please, Amy," he said. "I am fine. Please."

After unlacing and pulling off my snake boots, I stripped off the soggy pair of pants and flung them to the side while ants clambered

Chapter Twenty-Four

up my legs and bees swarmed all over the newly exposed skin. Eduardo and David swatted and knocked the creatures off of my body, while defending themselves at the same time, as I slipped on the dry, industrial green polyester and spandex Patagonia slacks.

For almost an hour, the fabric made me feel like a new person, decreasing the number of bees considerably. But as my sweat continued to pour, the moisture eventually seeped through every thread, saturating what I believed to be one of the best pairs of pants in the world. Before the bees increased further, the porters and trackers had packed up the area, extinguished the fire and were ready to move once again.

Besides the bees, there were other things I dreaded about the jungle. At the top of the list were the short periods of time when I was alone. Inevitably a bathroom break became necessary, which meant that I would need to venture into the jungle by myself. Being the only female, my quest for privacy was more out of respect for the others than any shyness.

While clearing multiple small areas to erect our tents early one evening, I realized that I could not hold it any longer—my bladder was full. Walking forty feet into the brush, I unzipped and partially dropped my pants and quickly urinated. But before I could walk back to the campsite, I felt multiple bites all over my upper body. Not knowing what it was, I began to slap my body with great force and yelled out to David, who was twenty feet away. As David hit my back, I continued to beat my arms and chest. And quietly moan.

Raising my shirt exposed large black ants, most of whom were dead. Apparently, in the few moments I had squatted to pee, they swiftly climbed up my pants and crawled inside my untucked shirt. David helped me pull off the bodies, their mandibles sunk deep into my skin. Within a couple of hours, the minor pain and discomfort from the bites had disappeared completely.

Campsites each night had to be chosen and prepared in the late afternoon because daylight disappeared quickly due to the thick canopy above. Clearing the tent sites with machetes took time, and the time gave ample opportunities for ants, bees and other insects to surround us in droves.

We had no choice but to endure while they covered our packs, bags, equipment and bodies. Always the first to arrive were various species of ants, which seemed to quickly overtake every article of clothing or object on the ground. The bees would arrive shortly thereafter, seemingly vying for any remaining space.

Our only escape in the evenings was to swiftly clear the areas, put up the tents and retreat inside as quickly as possible. But no matter how fast we unzipped and zipped the openings to our tents, insects always slipped in.

Inside the tent, I would take care of the few intruders before stretching out and watching the hundreds of others crawl and fly outside the tent's covering, only inches away. My headlamp shone brightly on the tent's canvas, and I watched in amazement the shadows of hundreds of constantly moving objects.

"This is unreal." I exclaimed one night to Eduardo and David, whose tents were within ten to fifteen feet of mine.

"I must have three to four hundred insects crawling on my tent now," David replied.

Chapter Twenty-Four

"Guys, do you want two packets of salmon or two packets of tuna with rice tonight?" Eduardo asked.

Laughing, I responded, "Can't we just stay inside and eat a Clif bar?"

After dark each night, when the numbers of bees diminished, we left our tents to boil water over the fire which would be used to cook rice. When the rice was ready, we would mix in two packets of either salmon or tuna. Our teammates instead preferred their own foods they had packed, which included more dried fish, often accompanied by a paste that was similar to peanut butter.

Because no one on the team ever complained, I looked closely when they had their shirts off for any concerning injuries, gashes or bites. The porters and trackers always responded as if there was no problem even when, in Western medicine, bandages or steri-strips were warranted.

Or when, like Eduardo and David, three of the porters were covered in numerous quarter-size whelps, which looked as if they were plagued with some dreadful disease. For David and Eduardo, we applied hydrocortisone cream. But the porters, although they were grateful, declined the treatment.

After the meals, inside the tents, Eduardo took care of the cameras and backup drives while David treated our water with SteriPens and reorganized the audio equipment that had been used during the day. I documented the day's journey in a small notebook and provided any bandages, medications, etc. that anyone needed.

I would then spread my saturated clothes across several waterproof bags in hopes that they would dry a little during the night. With high humidity, daytime temperatures in the eighties and nineties, and no direct sun, it was difficult for anything to dry during the day or night. Including our bodies.

On the first night in the jungle, six of us had draped our wet garments over tree limbs near the fire to dry, only to awaken the following morning to find every inch of fabric covered inside and out with ants and insects. We weren't sure if they were attracted to the damp clothing, the salt from our sweat or if our clothes had simply encroached upon their territory. Regardless, trying to rid the clothing of the inhabitants was not only frustrating, it also placed us at greater risk for bites and stings. The pain from a bite or sting was one thing, but if it led to an infection, severe reaction, parasitic disease or illness . . . that was quite another.

The truth is, I worried more about infection and parasitic diseases than I did snakes and large animals.

Each night, before going to sleep, I would take my headlamp and look at my body, surveying the day's damage. I had no idea the culprit to most of the marks that grazed my skin, and although my body was badly stricken with cuts and scrapes, red spots and blotches, whelps and streaks of dried blood, there was no intense pain or itching. Only minimal discomfort, like tenderness around a few of the bites and slight burning where the cuts were a little deeper.

The bites, scrapes and wet clothes didn't bother me that much. But my wet boots did.

As streams of sweat flowed down my body during the day, my socks became drenched, and tiny pools of water collected inside my boots. After the first day, the boots were never dry again. Each morning when I put them on, it took only a few moments before my clean, dry socks were soaked. Even though I had packed river sandals, I preferred the safety and protection of my Cabela's snake boots over their comfort, as did Eduardo and David.

The footwear of our teammates, however, varied between boots, sneakers and flip flops. Although Matoo originally had no shoes, he soon sported my new Vasque boots I had brought from the U.S.

Chapter Twenty-Four

Walking in wet socks created friction against the back of both heels and resulted in multiple large blisters. Bandages and skin coverings provided little relief, as they too became saturated and over the course of the day were gradually rubbed away. With each passing hour and day, the irritated areas worsened as the skin continued to peel, exposing an ever-increasing area of bleeding raw flesh.

Perspiration poured nonstop, and even though our bodies remained drenched in never-ending streams of sweat, the land itself was dry. Satellite images obtained by the Wildlife Conservation Society prior to entry had shown several streams and brooks along our route with which we could replenish our water supplies. But time and time again, the sources of water were nothing more than dry creek beds. Twice, porters went in search of water and returned hours later with brown water filled with sediment. On the third, fourth and fifth trips, they returned empty-handed.

After searching for days without success, there were only nine ounces of water remaining. We had no choice but to temporarily halt the expedition and exit the jungle. Resupply, regroup and recalculate.

We had gambled with finding water. And we had lost.

With every member of the team experiencing dehydration, we decided to exit the jungle by turning around and heading south. The southern border, we believed, was much closer than the northern border. Going west was actually the shortest distance to a logging road, but it would entail blazing a trail and possibly encountering difficult hurdles and dead ends. If we could at least follow parts of the course we had made on the way in, we would conserve energy by not having to chop and slash as much with the machetes while also allowing us to quickly cover more ground.

We could overcome the ants, bees, heat, thorns and briers. But we could not survive without water.

It was late in the afternoon when the decision to exit was made. It would be a long and difficult journey out, especially in weakened physical states. We would pitch camp earlier than usual each evening in order to allow more time to clear camp sites and have more time to rest. Food seemed to only exacerbate the thirst. So, during the next few days, very little food was eaten. A solemnness fell upon the group as even the porters and trackers were quiet at night—a behavior that was in deep contrast to the earlier nights in the trek with late-night loud talking and laughter.

In the darkness of each morning, we awakened, packed up the tents and continued on the journey south. The early morning hours gave a nice reprieve from both the bees and the intense heat.

With Matoo leading, the team followed behind as usual in single file. Headlamps and flashlights sent flickers and streams of light into the darkness, casting shadows that startled and spooked.

Matoo worked hard to stay on the path, but the route appeared one minute and disappeared the next. He searched for the markings on the tree trunks made by our machetes on the way in, and the branches and seedlings that the porters and trackers had broken and snapped, all of which served as markers for the path. But somehow, the jungle seemed not only to have hidden the signs—but devoured them.

The GPS rarely worked. The few times we received a signal were at points where large trees had fallen and created small openings in the canopy. The signals, when we did get them, were sporadic, weak and fleeting.

The compass was also unreliable. Twice, we had readings that conflicted with earlier readings. Donald speculated that it was the

Chapter Twenty-Four

earth of the Congo—maybe the minerals like iron which interfered. In Pokola, a friend of his who worked with the logging company warned him not to rely completely upon a compass.

Because of the limitations with the GPS and compasses, we had limited information on location. To lead us out we would continue to depend upon Matoo, in whom we had great faith . . . even though we had been lost several times in the days and nights prior.

The journey out was not easy. Dehydration was taking a serious toll. Sunken eyes, which seemed to age each of us ten years, screamed hopelessness and fear. Fatigue was so intense that it was hard to breathe and talk at the same time, while the body battled an ever-increasing number of falls, trips and stumbles, which required even more energy. And further slowed our pace.

Sweat continued to pour, and yet, I could not understand how we could be dehydrated and still sweat so profusely. It was becoming not only a tough physical challenge but also a psychological one. In order to climb over barriers and large fallen trees, we helped to lift each others' packs and bodies across the obstacles. The gestures alone seemed to bring hope.

Although I dreamed of the abundance of clear, clean water, I couldn't help but to fantasize further about the orange Fanta soda I would have when we returned to the village. Maybe two. I even thought of the ice-cold Red Oak beer I would eventually enjoy back home in North Carolina. A beer so cold it was uncomfortable to hold.

The fantasies temporarily distracted me from the realities, but the realities were never far from my thoughts.

Machetes slashed only when necessary, as conserving energy was paramount. Matoo ceaselessly scoured the surroundings for the path or for a better route. He was a natural navigator, veering right and then left, and then right again. His sense of direction was uncanny. I, on the other hand, could not figure out north from south, east from west.

On the day we projected we would exit the jungle, we packed up and left our make-shift tent site at five o'clock in the morning. After almost four hours of hiking, we came upon a large fallen tree that made a hole in the trees' canopy. The sky was clear, and the sun lit a small patch on the forest floor. Standing in the light, Eduardo pulled out the GPS and surprisingly got a signal. Holding it at arm's length toward the sky, he brought the device closer to take a look. He then turned to his right and held it high once more before drawing it close again.

"Shit," he exclaimed. "Amy!"

I quickly walked toward him while he continued to stare at the screen. Standing shoulder to shoulder, he pointed and then tapped his index finger on the apparatus.

In a solemn voice, he said, "We've been heading in the wrong direction."

Matoo had indeed began early that morning going south but had erroneously drifted west, then northwest and then north. For well over two hours, we had been going in the wrong direction.

The thick canopy made it impossible to determine the location of the sun, which would have given some guidance. We had no idea if the sun was to our right or left, in front or behind us. Without an active GPS, Matoo had been our best resource. But instead of heading toward the southern exit point, we were pushing back into the jungle's dense northern interior.

Chapter Twenty-Four

Donald relayed the discovery to Matoo, who appeared confused and frustrated at the news but didn't speak. There had been multiple times during the trek when he had become disoriented with direction. It was something that surprised him, Donald and the porters who knew him to be one of the best trackers around.

Then, Donald shared the news with the other members of the team. Immediately, they took off their packs and sat. They grumbled amongst themselves, and even though we could not understand their words, their demeanors spoke volumes. They shouted frustration. They cried defeat.

More than ever, we were in survival mode. The packs were heavy and burdensome, and we debated leaving contents behind to lessen the load, but the bags contained necessities. There was food that we needed for survival, tents and mosquito nets for protection, medical kits and machetes. And film equipment, of which Eduardo, David and I carried the bulk.

We knew our exit was going to be a difficult journey, to cover the distance we needed to cover in weakened states. But then, to have veered off-course so badly seemed to crush all hope.

I feared we would never find our way out.

I lowered my head and my eyes moistened as I thought of my partner, family and friends, fearing that I might never see them again. I berated myself for the expedition itself, an expedition that might lead to the deaths of nine others. And my own.

In silence, we sat.

After a few minutes, however, Eduardo stood and calmly spoke, "Come on guys. We can do this. Let's get out of here."

With his encouragement, everyone got up. It was a struggle to stand, and so taxing to pick up the packs that we had to help lift each others' packs to position them on our bodies.

Eduardo leaned over to David and me and whispered, "Guys, we have to keep moving. If we sit, we will only become more afraid. And give up. I don't want to die here."

I smiled and said, "Let's go."

"Let's get out of here," David reinforced.

Looking at the GPS once more through the opening of the fallen tree, Eduardo looked at Matoo and pointed south. With GPS held high, he picked up very infrequent and intermittent signals. And with them, he confirmed or corrected Matoo's course.

Twice, Matoo found paths made by forest elephants, which made our trekking much easier and increased our pace considerably. Even a small amount of water that had pooled in one of the elephant's footprints was collected and provided four to six ounces of water. The discovery lifted everyone's spirits.

Only when the elephant trails veered too far from our southern trajectory did we part from them.

It was getting to be late afternoon, and the team was relieved to pitch camp once again. Exhaustion had hit its peak, and depression seemed to linger alongside anxiety and fear. We passed around a couple of large ziplock bags of dried fruit, which the others didn't really like, but it seemed to be the only thing everyone could force themselves to eat. If only a bite or two.

Clearing the areas for the tents took great effort. Small trees and vegetation were only partially cleared, leaving protruding stumps and sharp edges that could easily pierce holes in the tents' fabric. But we didn't care. Even the bees and ants didn't bother us as much. We had more serious issues with which to deal.

The goal was to get the tents up as fast as possible, crawl inside them and rest.

The hours passed by quickly, and before we knew it, it was time

Chapter Twenty-Four

to pack up the site and move on. But the packing took a lot of time because of our limited energy and the need for frequent breaks. In time, we fell back into single file behind Matoo and Eduardo.

It was the day we prayed we would finally exit the jungle, and, like the other days, we hiked in silence. Until Donald stopped, pointed to a tree and spoke in his native language. Immediately, the porters took off their packs and walked the fifteen yards to the tree. With machetes, two of them cut the small tree into two-foot segments. Holding a segment into the air, a porter tilted his head back and opened his mouth to capture the water that flowed from the wood. And then passed it to the next man.

I looked at the end of the segment that was passed to me. It was solid, not the hollow center I expected. It was heavy and I struggled to hold it. But out of the solid mass dripped some of the most refreshing, clean water I had ever had.

Everyone had several swallows until the water was depleted from each piece. It was exactly what we needed. Physically and psychologically.

Several hours later, we finally made it to a logging road.

David dug into his pack and grabbed the satellite phone. Turning on the device, he walked several yards to his left before turning and walking a good distance to his right. But no matter the direction or distance, there was no signal . . . anywhere.

Without a signal, we could not call our drivers on standby. Without a call, no one knew to come for us. With no signal for the GPS, we had no idea how far away we were from the point where we had entered the jungle.

While David sought a signal, several porters walked down the road in search of a stream or water supply, believing that the logging road would at some point cross such a resource. Not long after they left, we heard Matoo's whistle.

Following his whistles, we soon discovered Matoo and the others standing half-naked in a small stream enshrouded by low-hanging branches. Its banks consumed by thick ground cover.

After filling our water bottles, we treated the contents with SteriPens before consuming bottle after bottle until we were satisfied. And then joined the others.

Our bodies seemed to instantly heal as the water both cooled and cleansed. It was the first time since we had entered the jungle that we had bathed. Its waters were shallow, only three feet deep, and our feet sank several inches into its squishy, muddy floor.

Initially, the mud was soothing and seemed to massage our blistered feet in its silky soft clay. But then I wondered about organisms that might dwell within the mud that we might be disturbing or other creatures in the water who found our arrival intrusive. Perhaps, too, it was the eerie silence of the spot, which should by all measures be teaming with life.

After ten minutes I left the water's embrace and climbed the stream's banks. Behind me, Eduardo followed.

I sat on one of the dry bags, grabbed one of the med kits and pulled out a tube of triple antibiotic cream, along with several bandages to treat the delicate places on the back of both my heels. The areas were tender and exposed, and I didn't want any infection. After cushioning the areas with additional bandages, I strapped on my river sandals. Eduardo also treated several areas of his body, including several deep cuts. We then left the supplies out for David, who remained in the water, to treat a plethora of spots on his body and for any member of the team, if they wanted.

Eduardo and I then filled our water bottles one more time and

Chapter Twenty-Four

grabbed a couple of protein bars from the food cache. We then unloaded our personal backpacks of backup drives and heavy camera equipment before placing the lighter weight packs on our backs and heading west in search of help.

David remained with the others as team leader. With him remained the satellite phone, three EpiPens and the GPS. Donald also remained with David to translate and to help manage the group in the event there was a problem.

Along every logging road were eco-guard stations. Since we had arrived in the country, we had stopped at many such stations where guards checked our passports, driver's licenses and vehicles and asked a multitude of questions: where we were coming from, where we were going, etc.

Because we didn't know our exact location, we had no idea how far away an eco-station might be. But since there was very little activity on the secondary road we believed we were on, if we simply sat and waited, it could be days or even weeks before anyone passed by.

The logging road was open and clear, without the protection of the forest canopy that blocked the sun and intense heat. Our river sandals and clothes quickly dried, only to be soon covered with the orange-red dust from the dirt road. Every step was painful with my blistered heels, but I didn't care. I was happy because we were all healthy, safe and hydrated. Plus, as long as we kept moving, we were free from the bees, which had begun to arrive in greater quantities at the stream.

Around every bend in the road, Eduardo and I hoped to find

a guard station. But time after time there was nothing more than another long stretch of road surrounded on either side by dense jungle. Finally, after walking over four miles, we saw a tiny building in the distance. Across the road in front of it was the single pole that served as the gate for an eco-guard station.

Our arrival startled the young man who sat inside the building, reading a book at a small wooden desk. Standing, he spoke a language we did not understand, almost as if to say, "Where did you come from?" Unable to understand each other's language, we used a form of charades to communicate.

Gesturing as if he had a phone next to his right ear, Eduardo repeated the words: "Phone, Pokola. *Merci*."

I held up eight fingers and pointed in the direction from which we came, attempting to communicate that there were eight others.

As the young man repeated Eduardo's gesture of holding a phone near his ear, he shook his head no. Then, walking around his desk, he held up a two-way radio and nodded yes. Speaking into the handheld microphone, he carried on a conversation in his language with a man whose words echoed throughout the room.

When the discussion was over, he grinned and said, *"Oui. Pokola,"* which meant 'Yes. Pokola' in French. Going back to our game of charades, he then acted like he was driving a vehicle and made the baritone sound of a large truck. Pointing to his watch, he lifted his index finger and said *"un,"* which meant 'one' in French.

"Oui," he said. *"Oui."* And then pointed to a bench, gesturing for us to sit.

A little over an hour later, a monstrous truck arrived, coming from the larger, northern logging road. The driver and his passenger climbed out of its cab as Eduardo and I followed the eco-guard walking toward the truck.

Chapter Twenty-Four

"*Merci*," we repeated to the guard and to the driver and his assistant. "*Merci beaucoup.*"

As I climbed the four steep steps to the truck's cab, I turned to look at its haul. A single tree. It was enormous; so huge that even at five-foot-seven-inches, I would easily have fit within its diameter. It was so massive it left no room for any others, protruding several feet beyond the sides of the truck and extending a good four feet beyond the tail of the truck's bed.

Seeing the massive tree initially brought sadness as I thought of how spectacular it must have stood within the forest. But then I remembered the conversation we had had with Donald on the day we scouted the entry point describing the low-impact logging practices. And thought how it must have been tagged and then cut.

Once inside the truck's cab, Eduardo and I thanked the driver and his co-worker in French once more and handed them a monetary gift. Eduardo leaned against the passenger door and dangled his right arm out its window. My body was closely sandwiched between Eduardo and the driver's assistant, who sat to my left. At the places where our bodies touched, sweat formed and dripped.

Turning on the ignition and putting the vehicle in gear, the driver powered the vehicle forward. For several hours, we barreled down the dirt road until we reached the logging facility, which was located on the outskirts of Pokola. It was as far as they were allowed to take us.

After thanking them once more, Eduardo and I walked another mile and a half before finally reaching the guesthouse, where we were greeted by Donileon. After making two phone calls, she finally located one of the drivers. Unable to find the second driver within twenty minutes, we decided to send the one available vehicle to pick up our team members.

And the Silent Spoke

Because there was only one vehicle, Eduardo and I remained in Pokola so that the eight remaining members could fit into the SUV. Along with the driver, we sent an abundance of clean water, Oreo cookies and slightly melted Kit Kats and Snickers, which we had stored at the guesthouse for the second part of the trek.

It was late in the evening when David walked into the guesthouse. Seeing him, I ran and hugged him.

I had never been so happy to see my friend.

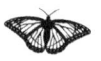

Chapter Twenty-Five

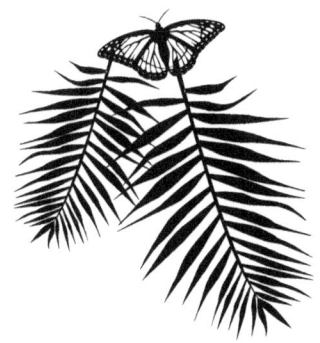

During the next two days in the village, we restocked supplies, reorganized and recalculated entry points for the jungle's northern region. According to satellite images from the Wildlife Conservation Society, the northern region had watering holes, and its terrain was more swampy than the southern territory. It would be unlikely that we would once again find ourselves dehydrated and without water.

Hopefully, it would also be free of the swarms of bees.

The jungle's northern edges were more permeable and less dense than those in the south. An entry point was quickly decided upon, and we ventured into the forest—single file behind Matoo—in order to chart the initial path we would follow the next day. Even though the terrain was relatively welcoming, the bees were not.

Their onslaughts seemed much worse than those we had encountered in the south, appearing in greater numbers and within shorter periods of time. Yet, it wasn't until Matoo, Hema, our driver and I emerged from the jungle ahead of the others, after blazing the beginnings of our trail, that we realized how much worse they really were.

And the Silent Spoke

When Matoo was only twenty feet from the SUV, he stopped suddenly and motioned for us to step forward and look. As we surrounded him on the narrow path, we stood still and in awe, staring at the thousands of bees blanketing our Land Cruiser. It was as if the vehicle was a huge hive.

Thousands of bees swarmed the exterior while hundreds more crawled and flew within the vehicle's interior. They flew in and out of open windows, covering bags and equipment and a pile of damp clothing that had been left behind.

Due to their tremendous numbers, it was impossible to simply shoo them out. So, we decided to drive them out. While the driver opened the driver's door, I opened the passenger door. When we did, many of the bees that were inside flew out. But others flew in. As he swatted the bees from his seat and steering wheel, I brushed others away from my seat and away from the gear shift.

In the back of the vehicle, one brave porter, Hema, opened the back doors wide, stepped inside and squatted amidst the swarms of the flying and crawling insects.

"Hema, are you okay? Are you good? Do you need to leave?" I asked while swatting away several bees, holding my thumb up and then pointing to the opened back door, knowing that he could not understand my English.

Raising his thumb, he nodded his head yes as he slapped away several bees encircling his head. Watching him, I ran my hand along my right-side pants' pocket, making sure the two EpiPens were secure.

With the windows down and the back doors wide open, the driver started the ignition and pushed the gas pedal to the floor, quickly shifting into second, then third and finally into fourth gear. Barreling along the dusty, narrow dirt road.

Chapter Twenty-Five

The air streamed through the windows into the SUV, creating great turbulence that seemed to grab the bees and thrust them into a spin, forcing them out the back of the vehicle. While the air carried most of them away, Hema and I used two damp socks to swat and expel the others.

When the majority of the bees were gone, the driver slowed, did a three-point turn and headed back. Seeing the others by the road in the distance, Hema and I hung out of the windows and yelled with excitement.

The territory of the northern jungle vibrated with a multitude of sounds. Birds, insects, monkeys. Several times, Matoo heard forest elephants that were within a hundred feet, but due to the thickness of the jungle, they remained out of sight. Other creatures were likely scared away by the constant slashing of our machetes.

In the evenings, it remained hot and humid, but inside the safety of our tents, there were no problems sleeping. Occasionally though, a noise would startle us awake. After reaching to my right and gripping the machete that lay only inches away, I would lie still, wondering what creature or creatures had made the sounds, while also trying to determine how close we were to one another.

With our tents in the midst of trees and dense growth, it was impossible to see far beyond a few feet, even with powerful headlamps.

Only once did we have the opportunity to camp in an area that permitted a view of the night sky. Through the hole in the canopy that had been created by the falling of several large trees, we gazed at a seemingly infinite array of stars dotting a perfectly clear sky.

It had been weeks since we had seen the evening sky. And stars.

To the right of where we sat by the fire was a healthy, gigantic tree whose trunk and branches seemed to reach for the stratosphere. Alongside it, slowly moving upward, from its trunk to its furthest limbs, was a bright yellow full moon.

"The moon's trajectory is straight up. I've never seen that," I said. "Do you think it's because we're so close to the equator?"

No one had an answer. And it didn't matter.

It was breathtaking.

The moments of beauty and peace helped to balance the challenges, especially with the bees. Although there were still swarms of what we believed to be honey bees in the northern region, there were also other species. With more elongated bodies and pointed heads, one species had stings that were more painful than the honey bees' and resulted in redness and swelling that lasted for hours. Knowing that the reactions would in time subside, we dealt with the stings and continued on.

That was, until Eduardo had a severe reaction to one of them. It was at that point that everything changed.

"Guys, I got stung," Eduardo said one evening while rolling up his right shirt sleeve. "It's not like the others. The swelling. It's tender. Painful, too. Not too bad, though."

Raising his arm, he pointed to a spot underneath his upper arm on his tricep and not far from his armpit. Surrounding the sting was an area of intense redness and inflammation—four inches and more in diameter.

"I kept thinking it would get better, but it's getting worse," he continued.

Pulling up his shirt sleeve further, I looked to see how far the swelling extended up his arm.

Chapter Twenty-Five

"Let's get fifty milligrams of Benadryl in you quickly and see if that'll help take care of the problem," I responded. "How are you feeling? Are you weak? Any difficulty breathing? Nauseated?

It's really hot. And swollen," I said as I wrapped my hands around his arm.

"Either the venom of these bees is more potent than the venom of the other bees . . . or your body has become sensitive and is having a hard time handling the envenomations.

Doesn't matter the reason. We have to take care of this.

"We have steroids, both oral and topical . . . Benadryl . . . and of course, the Epi as a last result. What are you thinking?" I asked.

As an EMT and wilderness survival expert, Eduardo responded as he had during every other serious situation on a trek . . . calmly. And practically.

"Let's do the Benadryl. That should do it," Eduardo replied.

Eduardo's reaction to the bee sting was similar to one that our porter Novi had experienced the day prior, which caused his right hand to swell two to three times its normal size. Seeing Novi's hand caught me off-guard; it was so puffy, the skin looked as if it could not possibly stretch any further and that at any moment it was going to burst.

Through translation, I asked Novi if he was having any other symptoms like difficulty breathing, dizziness or vomiting before asking if he wanted to take some of our medicine.

"He said he is okay and that it will soon go away. It has happened many times before." David and Donald translated. "He says to thank you."

I continued to check on Novi's hand throughout the next two days. Eventually the swelling diminished until his hand was nearing its normal size.

Eduardo's reaction, on the other hand, was only getting worse by the hour.

After Eduardo swallowed the Benadryl tablets, I took a black Sharpie marker and marked the outer edges of the redness and swelling. Over the next couple of hours we watched closely, hoping to see the redness and swelling retreat from the black markings. Instead, the swelling extended beyond the markings, pushing further down his arm toward his elbow and forearm.

Every four hours he took another fifty milligrams of Benadryl. New markings were made but the swelling continued beyond them as well. Raising both his arms with elbows bent, David and I compared the swollen right one to the normal left one.

"Dude—it's almost three times the size of your left one," David remarked.

"We are going to take care of this. Don't worry, Eduardo," I commented. "It could be worse. You could have had multiple stings. Or, God forbid, had a sting to your neck or face. And then gone to sleep without telling us.

Ohhhhh . . . Eduardo, that could have been really bad.

Sorry. I should not have mentioned that. You are going to be fine. David and I are not leaving your side."

I knew that if we remained with the swarms of bees in the area, it was only a matter of time before Eduardo or Novi, or possibly others on the team, experienced more of the same reactions. With only four EpiPens and only two medical personnel, the consequences could be devastating and deadly, especially if there were multiple life-threatening reactions at the same time.

Such a risk we could not and would not take.

After fourteen hours, the swelling with Eduardo's arm continued to expand beyond all black markings, forcing us to leave the

Chapter Twenty-Five

jungle and seek outside help. Luckily, Matoo knew the region well due to having family members in a nearby tribe.

"There's a clinic there." Donald and David translated the words Matoo spoke. "It's for the men who work for the logging company. And their families. But they will help us too."

Once we came out of the forest, it was a five-hour drive to reach the village and its clinic. There, a nurse did an initial evaluation on Eduardo, looking closely at his severely swollen arm.

"When this happens in the forest," she explained as Donald and David translated, "a person must immediately pull out the stinger and pee on the area. The urine will make it better.

You can also take ash from a fire, if it is available. Mix it with the urine and rub it on the site."

The thought of peeing on Eduardo's arm made everyone laugh.

"Everyone line up!" I joked.

"It must be *his* urine," the nurse laughed and pointed to Eduardo. "Only *his* urine will work.

But the urine will not work now. It has been too long. It is too late," the nurse continued. "We must see the doctor for medicine."

The doctor's office was a small thirteen-by-thirteen-foot room. In the far-left corner, a fan ran full blast circulating the humid, warm air. To the right, a lonely, wooden seven-foot-long shelf protruded from the wall, sparsely populated with a handful of worn medical textbooks and an old scale for weighing. On the opposite wall hung faded posters displaying prominently the letters HIV. Underneath their headings was smaller text written in a language I could not understand.

With a long, white lab coat and dark-rimmed glasses, the doctor sat at his desk. He looked up briefly when we entered and motioned for us to sit in the chairs facing him. He was handsome, in his mid-thirties, and on the desk in front of him, a stethoscope was draped over a pile of books.

His demeanor oscillated from that of a stoic academic to a gentle, empathetic caretaker. With David and Donald translating, Eduardo described the incident and the increasing inflammatory response while explaining the Benadryl that he had taken to help combat the reaction. As he spoke, the doctor checked his blood pressure and pulse.

"Bendrul?" the doctor asked.

"Yes," I answered, and David translated. "Fifty milligrams every four to five hours. Do you use it? We use it in the United States for allergic reactions. It is an antihistamine."

"Um . . . antihistamine," he responded as he walked over to the bookshelf and grabbed a medical textbook. Sitting back down behind his desk, he flipped through the pages and then turned the book around, facing us. And pointed.

Chlorpheniramine tablets 4 mg

"Yes. We use Chlorpheniramine as well. But we use Benadryl more often. It is also known as diphenhydramine. Do you know diphenhydramine?" I inquired.

The doctor, shaking his head no, slid the book toward me. I turned the pages and then searched the book's index for any documentation of diphenhydramine. But found none.

The doctor announced with translation, "I need to administer medicine. A steroid. It will help with the inflammation and will help the heart. The pulse is too fast."

"By mouth?" Eduardo asked as he mimicked putting a tablet in his mouth and chewing.

"Injection," Donald and David translated the doctor's response.

Leaning over and whispering, Eduardo asked, "Do you think

Chapter Twenty-Five

the needles are clean?"

"I'm not sure," I answered. "Let's see what he has."

The thought of an injection made both of us quiver. If the needle was not sterile, it could cause another problem. Or leave Eduardo battling something much worse . . . possibly for the rest of his life.

From behind us, the nurse walked around the side of the desk and handed two vials and an alcohol swab to the doctor. As she stood beside him, she tore open a package, pulled out a syringe and placed it on top of its ripped packaging in front of the doctor. Then, reaching over the desk, she took an old rubber tourniquet and tied it around Eduardo's arm.

In the meantime, the doctor took the syringe, injected it into one of the vials and slowly drew up a liquid diluent before inserting the diluent into the second vial containing the powdered steroid. After swirling and mixing the liquid with the powder, he inverted the vial, inserted the syringe back into the vial's rubber stopper and pulled out the solution.

Setting the vial down, he held the syringe out in front of him perpendicularly and thumped the top of its barrel several times to expel any air.

As he thumped the syringe, a thought flashed through my mind. Only months earlier, Eduardo had been given two rounds of chemotherapy, for which he had spent a week in the hospital. Although the oncologists fully supported his adventure to the Congo, they wanted him to take every precaution.

"Eduardo, the steroids—they may lower your immune system. Is this a good idea?" I whispered.

"I'm not sure, Amy," he replied. "And I'm not sure of that

syringe going in my body. I thought it was going to be in the muscle, not through my veins. Do you think it's okay?"

As we whispered, the doctor stuck the needle into Eduardo's arm. Standing up, I quickly reached across the desk, put my hand on the doctor's hands and said, "Please wait a moment."

With David and Donald translating, Eduardo explained that he had been given very strong medicines for cancer only months earlier and that we thought it was a good idea to ask his cancer doctor before he did the steroid. To which the doctor agreed. Reluctantly. And pulled out the syringe.

Because of the time difference, it was another eight hours before the oncologist's office was open. Speaking on the satellite phone, Eduardo explained the situation to his doctor in Ecuador. He told of the swelling and redness and the weak, rapid pulse.

Eduardo's oncologist felt the steroid shot was in his best interest, especially with the increased heart rate.

Returning to the clinic early the following morning, Eduardo apologized and asked if the doctor would administer the steroid. Smiling and nodding his head yes, the doctor opened another syringe, reconstituted another vial and injected the medicine.

Over the next twelve hours, the inflammation decreased considerably.

Although the reaction was under control and Eduardo's body was returning to normal, his reaction to the bee sting and the reaction that Novi experienced were enough to warrant an end to trekking within the jungle's deep northern territory.

With the decision, we said good-bye to the magnificent swath of forest we had spent weeks exploring. Both its southern and northern territories.

Chapter Twenty-Five

Both sections of the Congo jungle had not only been inhospitable, but intolerable. Not once did we cross paths with an indigenous person or even see signs of human life. Yet within its world void of mankind, the jungle birthed life that prospered and thrived.

And for a moment in time, we were immersed within its womb of diversity and wonder.

During those weeks, we walked upon virgin ground and breathed untainted air. We witnessed a world where the smallest of creatures had tremendous power and even dominance . . . and where humans wither.

We were overwhelmed by its complexity and humbled by its strength and expansiveness. And in the process, we glimpsed a purity and sacredness most endangered.

It was for many species, a pristine haven—rarely seen.

A flourishing ecosystem, existing perhaps as it has done so since the beginning of time.

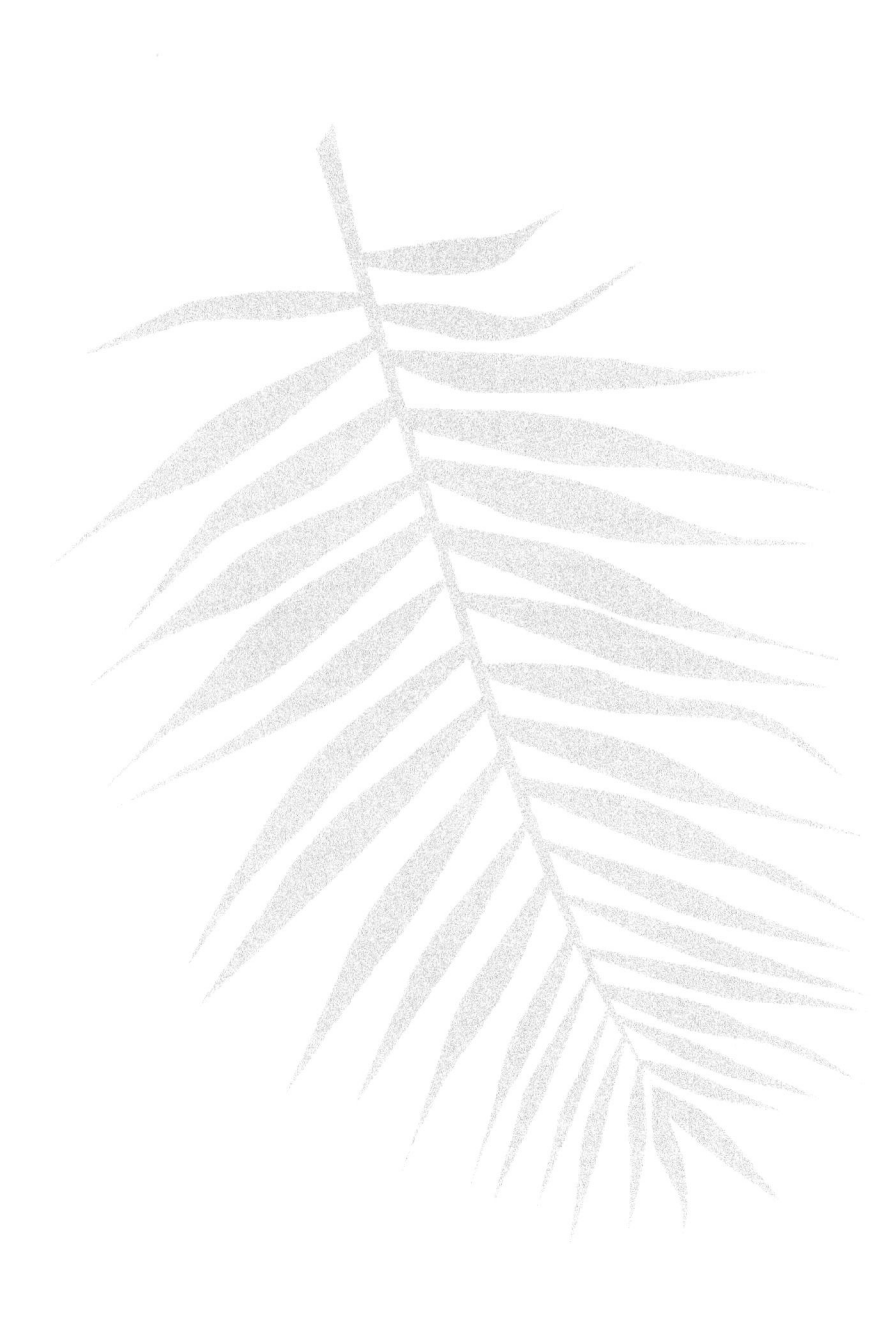

Chapter Twenty-Six

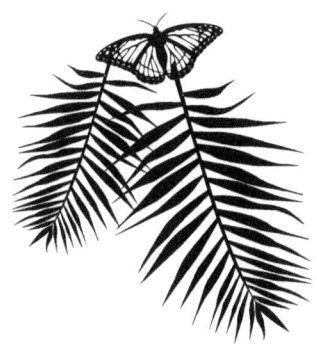

Taking a deep breath, she was surprised by a sudden strong scent of rubbing alcohol. The aroma was perplexing, as she couldn't recall if there was even a bottle of it in the home. Realizing that one of her nieces or nephews had likely just used it, she ignored the smell. And proceeded.

If Eduardo and David had not been with me, I'm not sure the jungle trek would have ever happened. Even though there were times when I was strong and persistent, there were also critical moments when I was not. Moments when my teammates' wisdom and strength not only propelled us forward but inspired me to see differently . . . and more clearly.

A person is lucky to have two, maybe three, true friends in life. Even luckier to have more. These are friends who are always there—who comfort when you walk through the deepest valleys and who celebrate when you reach the highest mountaintops. These are people who gently encourage you to broaden your perspectives and views, and who embrace you no matter the shortcomings.

Because of them, the deeper lessons of empathy, kindness, acceptance, love and forgiveness are often learned. Most of all, they, like an enduring partner or parent, rally you to be truthful to your soul . . . your passions, hopes and dreams.

She paused as Dominga came into the room and passed around a tray of homemade cookies and a pitcher of sweet tea.

My friendships with Eduardo and David remain close to this day. Over the years, my love and respect for them has only magnified.

Along with them, I've had other dear friends throughout life. Two of them, Shay and Dani, steered our post-production team for Healing Seekers. There was never a problem they felt could not be solved, or a goal that could not be reached. They reminded me that 'all is well'—and that hurdles, difficulties and defeats often lead to the greatest blessings.

Their optimism overflowed and their creativity poured, resulting in outstanding accomplishments—including several Telly Awards and International Film Festival Awards for our educational materials. Yet, it has been the friendship and the love we have shared that, to this day, make my heart sing.

Although age and distance have limited our interactions, the bonds of friendship with Shay, Dani, Eduardo and David have only grown stronger in these latter years of life. And more precious.

I know that God brought us into each others' lives for many reasons. I dare say that had it not been for the convergence of our individual passions, however, we may not have had anything more than a brief encounter in life.

And what a travesty that would have been.

At the right time, God brings together the right people. And it is because of those unions that we, as individuals, grow immensely, and are able to accomplish the things that often become the most meaningful in life.

Sighing quietly, she swallowed.
And pressed on.

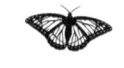
Chapter Twenty-Seven

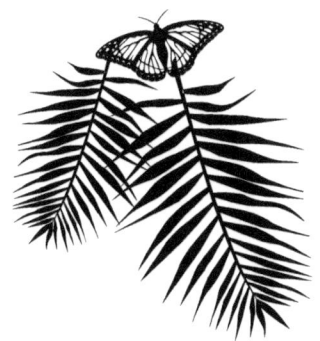

Leaving the jungle's northern region, we traveled northwest toward the upper reaches of the Sangha River. Located approximately sixty-five kilometers north of Ouesso and near the village of Matoo's family was a small village known to have a guesthouse. If we were permitted to stay, it would serve as our base camp for the next seven days.

The village was located along the eastern banks of the Sangha River. Across the river, on its western banks, was the country of Cameroon. Traveling the river further north, one would reach the Central African Republic.

Like every new region of the country in which we traveled and stayed, this area required a new set of permits and permissions that had to be obtained from the local authorities. Therefore, immediately upon our arrival into the village, we went in search of the local police authority and immigration officer.

A partially cleared hill separated the village from the forest. Scattered along the base of the hill were family huts and dwellings. Near the very top of the hill was an isolated thirty-foot-long wooden structure that served as the police quarters. Not far from it, on the side of the hill and hidden amongst trees, was an even smaller building known as the immigration office.

First, we sought permission from the police official, and then from the immigration officer. Each carefully reviewed our passports, film and research permits and asked a multitude of questions.

"Where are you coming from? What are you doing? Where are you going? How long are you staying?"

The men were focused and professional. And rarely smiled. With their approvals, we received stamped permissions and were granted our request to stay.

The guesthouse was located at the village's most northern edge. To reach it, we walked along a wide dirt path that went through the heart of the village. On either side of the path were small huts, often in a seemingly random zig-zag pattern. Outside several huts, women dipped garments in and out of wooden and plastic buckets filled with water. While children ran and played, the women washed and then spread the wet clothes upon the roofs to dry in the sun.

Walking five minutes further along the path, the huts all but disappeared. In their place, on either side of the trail, was brush and forest. Eventually we arrived at the guesthouse. A place we would call home for the next several days.

The guesthouse was a long, rectangular wooden building. At the far-left end, a red plastic cup floated in a large wooden barrel of river water. Donald explained that it was to be used for hand washing. Beside the barrel was a bright blue plastic gallon bucket sitting on the ground that was to be used for bathing in the wooden stall, forty feet away.

Inside, through the middle of the guesthouse, a long narrow hall permitted access to eight rooms. Each room was eight-by-

Chapter Twenty-Seven

twelve-feet and contained a thin mattress, mosquito net and a square wooden table. Directly above the table was a small opening cut into the wall, which functioned as a window.

Placing all of our bags inside the first room, Eduardo, David, Donald and I went to say good-bye to several porters and trackers who had fulfilled their jobs in the jungle and were departing our group to return to Pokola with our SUV driver.

With their departure, our team diminished to six. The members of our smaller team were Hema, Matoo, Donald, Eduardo, David and myself.

Outside the guesthouse, we hugged and shook hands, thanking each of them while paying them more than we had agreed upon. Eduardo set up one of the cameras on a tripod in order to take a group photo—something that we had not done during all of our weeks together.

Before he could snap the picture, however, the police official who we had met an hour or so earlier screamed from a distance. Following closely behind him were two other officers.

As Donald translated the officer's words to French, David translated them to English.

"He says we're in violation of the law. What the crap?" David exclaimed.

As the officers came closer, the chief officer continued yelling while pointing to the camera on the tripod.

David continued, "He keeps saying 'violation!'"

When they were within a few feet of our group, Donald and the officer went back and forth in a heated discussion. Intermittently, Donald translated the words for David.

"He wants to see all that we have," David translated. "He is demanding that we take him to our rooms and show all our belongings.

He is saying we are in violation of the law.

Guys—Donald is mad. Really mad! He says the officer is just wanting to cause a problem."

While the yelling continued, Donald reached into his shirt pocket and pulled out a copy of the filming permit. Holding it out, he extended it to the officer, explaining that we had a permit to film. The same permit he had seen only an hour or so earlier. But the officer ignored the outstretched paper and instead turned his back to Donald and walked toward the entry door to the guesthouse.

Only steps behind, Donald followed the officer, begging him to look at the paper, explaining that we had permits . . . that there was no violation. But the officer continued to ignore him.

Behind Donald, the rest of us followed into the guesthouse. Inside, the officer stopped and made a firm sweeping gesture with his right hand toward the rooms down the hall, demanding Donald show him the rooms with our belongings.

With his head down, Donald stepped in front of the chief officer and led him a few feet down the hall into the one room where we had quickly placed all our belongings. The room was so small and the bags and pieces of equipment so numerous, that even straddling the objects on the floor gave little room for the head officer, Donald and David to stand.

Eduardo and I, in the meantime, stood within the doorway as the officer continued with raised voice and Donald continued his pleas.

So intense was the situation that Donald rarely took time to translate, and when he did, it was brief. David, in turn, translated the fragmented sentences, most of which made little sense and left us more confused.

"He thinks we are reporters . . . something about trying to spy on them. I'm not sure," David translated. "He wants to go through

Chapter Twenty-Seven

all of our bags to see what we have. Equipment, cameras, computers, everything.

Donald says the guy is just wanting to cause a problem. And to show his authority."

For the next hour, the officer looked inside each bag, pack and container. Many of the bags, he only peeked inside, but others, he rummaged through clothing, food, equipment and supplies, pulling out items, flinging and scattering them on top of the mattress and across the room. When he finished inspecting one bag, Eduardo and I would step into the clutter, grab the bag, stuff as much of the contents back inside and place it in the hall so that he wouldn't go through it again.

During the process, the officer pulled out backup drives, med kits, waterproof containers, the satellite phone and receptor, and so on. He tried to open and pry apart and even shake items while asking: "What is this? What is in here? Why do you need this?"

When he got to the drone cases, he demanded Donald to open them.

"What is this?" He exclaimed, with widened eyes.

The moment Donald said, "drones," the officer went ballistic.

"He is saying it's espionage!" David translated from Donald. "That we have come to spy.

He—he's saying we are going to jail!"

With fury, the officer then ordered his two subordinate officers, who were standing in the hallway, to take us to jail. With the command, Donald pulled out the piece of paper that was our filming permit and angrily spoke to the officer, insisting that he look at the permit, which allowed the drones and cameras.

Puffing his chest out, the officer extended his arm so that the palm of his right hand was within inches of Donald's face. He then yelled and demanded that Donald shut up.

Stoically, the officer turned and motioned for us to follow as he stormed out of the room, down the hall and exited the guesthouse—charging toward the dirt road. Behind him, our team followed. Behind us, his two subordinate officers.

Like a herd of sheep, we trailed the chief officer, walking back through the village and past the huts until we were once again in the small building known as the police quarters.

We had been in the village less than three hours.

The station's vantage point at the top of the village's main hill allowed visibility of much of the village. Located in the front, far-right corner of the building were three steps that led to a narrow thirty-foot-long porch. Near the opposite end of the porch was a door, which led inside.

Five feet inside the door, a single wooden desk sat in the middle of the room. Directly in front of the desk and against the wall was a four-foot-long seat, part sofa and part bench. On it, the three of us and our head guide Donald were told to sit.

Because there were no other seats, our teammates who were porters and trackers were told to line up and stand against the wall. The chief officer took his seat behind the desk while his two subordinates stood close behind him.

I breathed deeply . . . and thought, here we go again.

The chief officer spoke loudly. Although he refused to let us speak, he did allow for translation.

But the necessary double translations took time. For which the officer had little patience. Before Donald could finish translating the officer's words to French, the officer would start talking again.

Chapter Twenty-Seven

When he did, Donald stopped in order to hear what he was saying.

David received only fragmented statements and half-sentences.

The officer's constant interruptions were further exacerbated by his rudeness in raising his voice when Donald attempted to translate, making it more difficult for David to hear, much less understand what Donald was saying. Even though Donald sat only inches away.

"We are in trouble. Something about the drones and equipment. I can't understand," David frantically whispered.

Eduardo and I responded, "Why? What did we do? We have permits. Can we make a phone call? Can we call the Colonel?"

By the time we would get a question back to David, he was being nudged by Donald, who would get a few more words translated before he was drawn back to the officer's commanding voice.

The three languages jumbled so that at times there was nothing but a bunch of incomprehensible words. The chaos and babble of the various languages, with its lost information and questionable understandings, went on for over two hours. When it finally subsided, the only thing that was clear was that we were being charged with espionage.

"I can't believe this is happening again," Eduardo sighed.

"This is crazy. This guy doesn't want to listen. He won't even acknowledge the permit!" David relayed.

"Donald looks worried. And scared. This is not good." I added.

"Remember when I spoke with the U.S. Embassy right after the first arrest? He said there's heightened sensitivity in the country with cameras, due to the upcoming presidential election. Remember when he mentioned the Al Jazeera news team that was asked to leave the country after only being here a few days?

We need to stress that we are not reporters or a television news team."

Through David and Donald's translations, we reiterated that we had the proper permits to film and that we were filming for educational purposes. At the same time, we emphasized that we were not news reporters and that our work was not politically related.

Finally, the chief officer agreed to look at the film permit. While he did so, Donald continued to fiercely defend our right to have the cameras and drones.

Pointing to each line on the paper, which was written in French, Donald translated the permit for the officer. He pointed firmly to the signatures of government officials at the bottom of the page, and to the stamp that the officer himself had given earlier in the day, acknowledging its validity.

After staring at the paper a few more minutes, the officer looked up. And agreed to let us go.

As we walked down the hill away from the building, I turned and looked back. Standing on the porch, leaning against its railing, was the head officer and his two subordinates. Watching us.

A sinking feeling came over me, much like I felt after the first arrest in Pokola. But this time, for reasons I could not fully grasp, there was an even greater amount of anxiety and trepidation. It seemed no matter what we might do in the next few days, they were going to be watching our every move.

Returning to the guesthouse, we said our final goodbyes to our teammates as they loaded into the SUV to return to Pokola. Sadly, we did not risk taking a group photo.

The incident with the police not only brought a level of stress and frustration, it also stole a chunk of time that had been set aside

Chapter Twenty-Seven

for a visit with a nearby healer. Returning to the guesthouse, we grabbed the cameras and day packs and went in search of the Baka healer, whom the owner of the guesthouse had told Donald about upon our arrival.

The Baka were hunter-gatherers, and the village was known to be home to a kind, gentle and joyful tribe. Their dependence upon the forest included using its natural resources for medicine and healing.

To reach the Baka village, we walked back through the village where we were staying and passed the police station before veering off onto a narrow, overgrown path. The ground cover consumed the faint markings of the trail while thick brush and trees hovered around and above it, making the path difficult to follow.

With Matoo leading and cutting back much of the foliage with his machete, we ultimately emerged from the woods to find a small cleared area surrounded by four tiny huts. Beyond the four huts were others that had been built along the edges of the surrounding forest. While we waited at the outskirts of the cleared area, Donald walked into the village to ask permission for us to visit.

Minutes later, he returned with an elder. Possibly in his fifties, he wore a ragged pair of brown shorts and a ripped white T-shirt. Vibrant and spunky, he walked swiftly beside Donald. Donald stood at least two feet taller than the elder. For every step Donald took in his flip-flops, the elder took two in his bare feet.

Making a direct path to us, the elder smiled and eagerly shook each of our hands.

I liked him immediately.

A few minutes later, a second elder from the village appeared. Much like the first elder, he had a small stature, standing not much more than four feet in height. Leading him by his arm was a younger man.

And the Silent Spoke

When they got within a few feet of where we stood, the young man spoke to the second elder, released his arm, and took several steps back. When he did, Donald grabbed the second elder's hand and shook it before making introductions.

The elder smiled, squinting to the point that his eyes remained almost closed. I could not tell how much he could see or could not see. Only that he had difficulty.

"His name is Lakuneta," David said as he translated Donald's words. "He is the village healer."

"Ahhh," I responded as I embraced and shook his hand with both of mine. Feeling my hand, he grabbed it tightly and smiled.

"It is an honor to meet you," I said, while David and then Donald translated. "Thank you for allowing us to be with you. And to visit your village."

"Hmmmm hmmmm," Lakuneta responded as he grinned.

"Where are you from? What brings you here?" Lakuneta asked as Donald, and then David, translated.

"We are from the United States. It is a place far away, across the ocean. We flew on a plane for many hours. My home is a place called North Carolina.

We have traveled such a long way because your way of life is very interesting to us. How you survive, how you heal if you are sick or injured . . . the beauty and history of your tribe. And your land.

We film with cameras, if you allow, and then we are able to show other children and people in the world who have never seen your village, culture and ways of life."

"Hmmm," Lakuneta responded before speaking further.

Donald then turned, nodded his head yes and said, *"oui."*

While Lakuneta spoke, Donald frequently asked Matoo, who was also a member of the Baka tribe, to verify that he was understanding the healer correctly.

Chapter Twenty-Seven

Unfortunately, soon after the conversation began, daylight started to disappear. Donald suggested that we head back to the guesthouse so that we would not get lost on the trail, especially since we had not packed headlamps.

Due to the incident with the police, we had lost many hours that we had anticipated spending with the village. Because we wanted to spend more time with Lakuneta, Donald recommended that we ask the healer if we could return in two days. Two days, because the next day Donald had arranged for a boat to take us up the river to visit other villages.

Lakuneta agreed, stating that he was happy we would return.

Shaking hands once more, we departed the healer and his village and headed to the guesthouse.

That evening, the wife of the owner of the guesthouse graciously prepared a dinner of fresh fish, rice and yucca dough balls. Afterwards, Eduardo, David, Donald and I rinsed off and went to our separate rooms. Although I was physically and emotionally tired, it was difficult to sleep. Rats scurried, and I was unable to determine if they were inside or outside the room . . . or within the walls.

Sliding out from underneath the mosquito net, I rummaged through my dry bag, opened one of the med kits and grabbed an alcohol swab which I opened, unfolded and used to clean my hands and feet. Back inside the confines of the mosquito net, I double checked to make sure no part of my body was pressing up against the netting, especially my fingers.

During our treks in Papua New Guinea, we had been warned multiple times to make sure that food, or the scent of food, was never left on our hands before going to sleep. Rats would come during the night, especially when we were on the Sepik River, and nibble on anything with even the faintest aroma of food. Babies and children often awakened crying from the rats biting their unprotected bodies.

Turning on both my headlamp and flashlight, I positioned them so that the beams covered my body, hoping that the light would deter any creature from coming close. I'm not sure if it made a difference, but psychologically, I felt safer.

The room was hot, and the only ventilation was through the small window a couple of feet away. Before I had crawled under the mosquito net, I had pushed back the two wooden slabs that served as shutters, allowing the rare breeze to enter the room. Although the moments were infrequent and brief, the air refreshed and cooled the room as well as my body.

The opened window, however, also allowed a variety of flying and crawling insects and creatures to enter. Throughout the night they could be heard often inches away, buzzing and flittering on the other side of the mosquito net.

The next morning, Donald left close to sunrise to go into the village to buy eggs. He found an older man who provided not only fresh eggs but also a loaf of hot baked bread from an outside clay oven.

As our team gathered outside, the guesthouse owner's wife heated water over a fire and poured it into cups containing the black grounds of instant coffee. As we sipped the coffee, she cracked open the eleven eggs Donald had purchased, placed them into a dented black pan, and scrambled them.

Chapter Twenty-Seven

After breakfast, we grabbed our day packs and left for a full day on the river.

Our boat driver was a young man in his early twenties, born and raised in the village. Wearing a torn pair of dark blue shorts, he waited in the boat at the bank's edge, barefoot and shirtless.

Seeing us, he waved and then turned to walk to the back of the boat, where he pulled the cord to the outboard motor. With the motor running, he motioned for us to board.

The river was quiet. Beyond the splashing water along the sides of our dugout, there were only the sounds of insects and birds greeting the day.

Along the banks, trees and vegetation were so thick and abundant, they seemed to morph into one giant entity. Various shades of brown and green swirled and spotted the landscape for as far as we could see. Trees towered as if climbing toward the firmament while their understories appeared to occupy every space below. Where the land met the river, limbs grew in a downward curvature, much like the rib of an umbrella, reaching out until they touched the water.

Two hours into the trip, our driver steered the boat toward several fishermen who were standing on a sandbar that jutted out from a piece of land near the border with Cameroon. Donald made a brief introduction and explained our interest in the local cultures, their ways of life as well as their healing remedies and rituals.

One of the fishermen stepped forward and came within a foot of Donald to speak further. He was a young man in his early twenties with widely spaced eyes and hair neatly trimmed along his hair line. His smile exposed beautiful white teeth, which had a considerable gap between his two front incisors.

Pointing up the river, he announced that his village was an hour or so further, toward the Central African Republic.

"His name is Divin," David translated from the words Donald spoke. "He's going to show us a plant . . . maybe it's a few plants, I can't tell . . . that his village uses."

As David spoke, the young fisherman turned inland and motioned for us to follow. A steep six-foot embankment separated the sandbar from the forest. To scale it, Divin climbed a crafted wooden ladder that had been placed at a thirty-five-degree angle. Made from tree limbs tied together with vines, the ladder was knobby and wobbly and gave slightly with each step. Without anything to hold onto, it took great balance to walk erectly across its rungs.

Into the forest Divin led our small group, slicing through limbs and plant growth with his machete until he stopped and placed his hand on the trunk of a tree, the diameter of which was two and a half feet. Above him were the outstretched limbs of the tree, covered in leaves that were bright lime green.

As Divin spoke and Donald translated the words to French, David shared them in English.

"This tree he uses for pain," David said. "When you have pain . . . hold on . . . I'm not understanding this.

Douleur. Où est la douleur? Quel genre de douleur?" David asked Donald in French.

"Ohhh," David continued. "He says it is for areas that are hidden. The bark is used for urination, but it also sounds like it's for sexually transmitted diseases. Diseases for the man.

Sounds like it's common here."

"Oh," I said. "Will you ask how often they give this and for how long at a time? Does it heal the problem completely . . . or is it something a person must take for the rest of their lives?

Chapter Twenty-Seven

And one more—is this only for men? Or for women too?"

As soon as the questions were translated, so too were the answers.

"He says it's taken three times a day for maybe two weeks. It takes care of the problem. But, a person sometimes reinfects themselves, and if they do, they will have to take it again. It is mainly for the men who have the diseases. But a woman may take it too."

Excited, Divin picked up his machete, which he had jabbed into the ground beside him, turned and walked further inland. Until he stopped at a second tree.

"This one," David translated to Eduardo and me, "is for severe injuries like deep cuts—gashes—like accidents by a machete. He said you can use this even if the arm is almost cut off. Wait a minute, let me make sure that's what he said.

Avez-vous dit que vous pouvez l'utiliser si le bras est presque coupé?" David asked Donald.

"Yep." David continued, "He said it is used for really bad cuts and accidents. The bark stops the bleeding . . . heals the wound completely."

With his machete, Divin stepped closer to the tree and chopped off a piece of the tree's outer bark and flung it into the woods. Squatting, he then picked up a large green leaf and, cupping it in his hand, stood and placed it against the tree, near the bottom of its newly exposed area. Taking his machete, he scraped the freshly cut area until half a cup of its shavings had fallen inside the leaf.

"The shavings need to be put in the sun to dry. You have to dry it thoroughly," David translated. "Once it's dry, you pack the wound with the shavings and cover."

"What do they use to cover it with?" I asked.

Patting his left forearm with his right hand and making a motion as if he was tying something around his forearm, Divin answered.

"They take fresh leaves and lay them on top of the shavings," David translated, "Then they wrap small vines around the leaves . . . which hold the leaves in place."

As I listened, I wondered how he knew such things. What caused the first person to scrape the inner bark of the tree? Dry it and then place it inside raw flesh? Why didn't the wounds become painful and infected?

When I asked how he learned of such medicine, the only answer Divin gave was that the remedy had been passed from his grandfather's father to his grandfather to his father. He had no idea how it began or how anyone learned of it.

And it didn't matter.

What mattered was that it worked. And had done so for generations.

Leaving Divin, we reloaded the dugout and continued north. During the course of the day, we spent time in two villages. The healers and villagers were generous and kind, gracious and inviting, even though our visits were unexpected. We learned about treatments for stomach aches and toothaches, infections and malaria.

Along the way we also met the chief over all the local villages.

"What is the greatest threat to your villages?" I asked after sitting with the chief for over an hour. "Is it tribal fighting . . . food . . . disease?"

"He said it is sickness," David translated. "Sickness that comes quickly. Things they don't know how to treat . . . and spreads quickly from tribe to tribe. Many die. Men, women and children."

Chapter Twenty-Seven

It was late afternoon when we boarded the dugout and turned south in order to return to the guesthouse. We would make only one more stop.

One of the men we had met earlier in the day told Donald that on our way back to the guesthouse, there was a point in the river where the water is shallow from the banks of Cameroon to the banks of the Congo. Along this path, elephants cross most days in the late afternoon.

Not once during the expedition had we seen one of the magnificent creatures, even though we had walked the paths they had made and dodged their piles of poop while we trekked in the jungle. Eager to see them, we beached the boat on a narrow sandbar, half a mile downstream from the crossing. With cameras and drones in hand, we watched and waited.

The area was quiet and still. An hour passed. But there was not one elephant in sight. We flew the drone over the jungle's canopy and along the river, hoping to find them and follow their common migration.

As the second hour slipped away, daylight also began to disappear. And with it, our dreams of ever seeing the creatures in the Congo. Eduardo held out a remaining hope, however, and asked Donald to remain a few minutes more. And a few minutes more. Until Donald finally insisted we leave.

Pushing off the sandbar, our boat driver started the motor and headed back to the village. It was almost dark.

I looked at Eduardo, who was fidgeting with one of the cameras. Although he didn't say a word, I knew he was terribly disappointed. Since the first day of the trek, he had spoken of photographing the

And the Silent Spoke

elephants. The crossing was perhaps the last opportunity we had to do so.

Grabbing my backpack, I pulled out my headlamp, notebook and pen and began to document the day's events. For almost two hours, we traveled the river in darkness. By the time we neared the village, we were tired, dirty and hungry, so as soon as the boat was pulled onto shore, all of us, including the boat driver, grabbed the equipment and packs and began the twenty-minute walk to the guesthouse.

The path from the river to the village was eight feet wide, and its sides were covered in four-foot-tall vegetation. Even though it was partly cloudy, there was an abundance of stars illuminating the sky.

Suddenly, the quiet was disrupted by loud voices coming toward us. Seeing the group of fifteen to twenty individuals in the evening was surprising, especially near the river. The closer the group came, the louder and more boisterous their yells.

In front of the group was the same chief officer that had originally granted our request to stay and who also marched us to the headquarters the day before. On his either side were his two subordinate officers.

In his right hand, the chief officer held what looked to be a homemade sawed-off shotgun. Raising it into the air, he yelled and shook the gun with intensity at us. The closer they got, the more obvious that the angry yells were directed at us.

"Donald! Donald! What's going on? What the heck? What is he saying? What did we do?" Eduardo, David and I clamored.

Donald was panicking. With a stunned look, he shook his head left to right and back again while answering.

David translated, "He doesn't know . . . he doesn't know. He's only saying that something is very wrong."

Chapter Twenty-Seven

While madly waving the weapon in the air, the officer stormed toward us. The closer he came, the louder his yells and the rowdier and more obnoxious his followers.

When he was within a few feet of our group, he turned and walked directly to our boat driver. With the gun raised high into the air, he cocked his arm back and then slammed the gun's stock into the back of the boat driver's head, causing him to suddenly go limp. His knees hit the ground as his body flung forward, catching himself only moments before his head hit the ground. With soft moaning, he struggled to get into a kneeling position. There he remained, grabbing the back of his head.

Gasping, I exclaimed, "Shit!"

"What the hell is going on, Donald?" David demanded.

"What the fuck is going on? What did we do?" Eduardo followed.

"Je ne sais pas. Je ne sais pas. Je ne sais pas!" Donald responded with eyes wide open.

"He has no idea!" David replied.

While we frantically whispered to one another in the darkness, the officer continued to yell and scream in his native language.

Donald's usual strong and confident demeanor vanished and in its place was the behavior of a frightened child. Like the rest of us.

Even when we insisted that Donald translate and explain what was happening, he remained in a quiet stupor. As if in a state of shock.

After the officer continued his tirade for several more minutes, he turned and commanded that we follow. With help, our boat driver got to his feet, and together we walked behind the officer. His two subordinate officers and the group of supporters, meanwhile, gathered behind us, berating and prodding us like a herd of cattle.

While we walked, Donald relayed what little he could decipher. That we were in lot of trouble. That we had broken the law. That we were all going to jail.

"Why?" David asked.

"What did we do?" I questioned.

"Guys, no one knows where we are. We need to call the Colonel. Now!" Eduardo replied.

Our satellite phone, however, was in one of the dry bags. To retrieve it, we would need to stop, open the bag and pull it out. Fearful that the officer's rage would result in another injury or worse, we decided we had no choice but to wait and get it later.

My mind raced. Had we flown the drone over a government occupation? Too close to the bordering country of Cameroon or the Central African Republic?

At the police quarters, we entered the same room, and once again, Donald, David, Eduardo and I were told to sit on the same sofa bench. To our left, Matoo, Hema and our boat driver were told to stand against the wall. In the door's entry way stood the two subordinate officers.

The chief officer alternated sitting and standing behind his desk, yelling and pounding his fist onto the desk. He shifted his focus from Donald to David to me and then to Eduardo before repeating the same circuit. When Donald attempted to translate, the chief officer went ballistic, demanding silence.

After close to thirty minutes, Donald was allowed to translate.

"We are being charged with traveling on the river after dark. And espionage." David translated Donald's words. "We are being called criminals . . . and must be punished. Donald is terrified. This is not like the other arrests. This is much worse."

"What? We have permits. We didn't do anything wrong!" Eduardo and I responded.

But before we could say anything more, the officer interrupted and commanded silence so that he could continue his verbal floggings.

Chapter Twenty-Seven

The chief's fury was terrifying. In a great exhibit of anger and to demonstrate his power, he brazenly thrust his gun into the air before shaking it at us. At times when he stood, he leaned far across the desk causing us to spontaneously physically withdraw.

With his close physical presence came the shocking faint smell of alcohol.

Our first arrest in Pokola weeks earlier had been horrifying. Yet it seemed to somehow pale in comparison to this. Verbal reprimands were one thing, but when they were combined with rage and violence . . . and weapons . . . it became quite another. Fear turned to paralysis.

After hours of intense verbal lashings in a language we did not understand, the chief ordered that we submit all of the belongings that we carried. Every bag, pack, camera and piece of equipment. It would be confiscated and then all of us would be placed in jail.

As we handed over the bags, he pointed to the necklace around Donald's neck. The necklace was a gift from his wife. It was a symbol of their love . . . Donald's most cherished material possession.

Donald refused to take it off. He begged the officer as he spoke of his wife. But no matter how hard he tried, the officer was relentless, ultimately insisting that Donald place the piece of jewelry in his outstretched hand. Fighting back tears, Donald lowered his head and slowly slipped off the necklace, placing it in the open palm of the officer's right hand.

With the necklace in his hand, the head officer motioned for one of his two subordinates to come to him. After whispering for a few minutes, the deputy officer motioned for Hema, Matoo and our boat driver to go inside a small room ten feet away. Once they were inside the room, the subordinate officer slammed the door and began yelling.

The chief officer then turned to us and resumed his inquiry while carefully going through each backpack. Each dry bag. Each equipment case. Just like earlier, but more meticulously.

One by one, items were placed on his desk as he documented on a white sheet of paper the contents. During the process he came across our three small bundles of cash, the sum total of which came close to one thousand U.S. dollars. A considerable amount of money for most people in the country. Each time he discovered one of the bundles, however, he handed the money to us so that we kept it in our possession. His actions both surprised and baffled us.

As he sorted through our possessions, Eduardo, David and I whispered to one another in English.

"We need to get in touch with the Colonel," Eduardo said.

"Yes. And it wouldn't hurt to also call the Ambassador," I mentioned.

"And Denise!" David added.

Addressing the officer in charge, David spoke in French while Donald translated to the officer's language, asking if we could make a phone call.

"S'il vous plaît, pouvons-nous faire un appel téléphonique?" David asked.

Donald's translation caused an outburst from the officer. Followed by another ten minutes of yelling.

"Damn," David said. "He won't let us make ANY phone call! He wants all our phones on his desk now! Our personal cell phones—the satellite phone . . . everything.

Anything we use for communication.

He also wants our passports.

We are screwed."

Chapter Twenty-Seven

Because our itinerary had changed only days earlier when we needed to leave the jungle's northern territory because of the bees, no one knew where we were. In fact, if we failed to return to Ouesso or to the USA as scheduled, any search parties would be focused in the jungle, not in the village or even in the region where we now found ourselves trapped.

When the officer completed his inspection of our belongings, we were allowed to speak. As with the other incidents, we apologized repeatedly for anything we had done wrong, explaining that we intended no harm or disrespect. We explained our work with filming as we presented once again the permits to do so. But no matter what we said, the officer was fixated upon a guilty verdict.

The officer then pushed his chair back and stood. And directed us to the side room where the other two porters and boat driver had been taken earlier.

The room was empty of furnishings. Along the far wall, Matoo, Hema and the boat driver stood, frightened and speechless, staring at us. Once we were all inside, the chief slammed shut the door, leaving the seven of us alone in the room.

With Donald and David translating, we asked if they were okay.

"They have been interrogated and threatened," David relayed. "The officer was trying to find a discrepancy between what we are saying and what they are saying. The officer wanted to see if we were lying, or if they would confess that we had done something illegal.

As Matoo and Hema spoke, they became teary, fearing that they were going to jail . . . to be locked up. Never to see their families again.

I looked at Donald, who stood to my right. Lowering his head, he wiped a tear with his right thumb from the corner of his eye. Although he was the strongest and toughest man I had met in the country and always seemed to be in control, he now appeared hopeless and powerless.

Whispering amongst ourselves, we tried to understand all that had taken place and all that was taking place. But we could not understand why we were in such trouble. We ruled out the notion it was for money, as the chief officer insisted that we keep possession of our cash. We had the correct permits for filming and had gone through the appropriate channels for entry into the village, which the chief officer had personally approved.

Although we were afraid of spending a night in jail, it was the thought of being locked up for an extended period of time, or indefinitely, that elicited indescribable panic.

After almost an hour, the chief officer abruptly opened the door and motioned for us to return to the main room.

With Donald translating the chief officer's words to David, David relayed the words in English.

"He says the three of us can return to the guesthouse. But we have to come back in the morning. At sunrise. Everyone else has to stay in jail because—it sounds like—they knew better."

As if a death sentence, soft moans spontaneously erupted as Matoo, Hema, Donald and our boat driver bowed their heads in defeat. Eduardo, David and I begged the officer for the opportunity to pay whatever fines were needed for our friends' release, insisting that they were only doing their jobs, helping us with our work. And should not be punished.

But no matter how hard we tried, the chief officer shook his head no and refused. Finally, Donald insisted that we leave and leave quickly, before the chief changed his mind and put us in jail too.

Chapter Twenty-Seven

It was very difficult to leave knowing what each of our teammates might face. After our first arrest, we had heard horror stories of assaults and beatings of those in jail. Stories that would make a person cringe.

Before leaving the room, we hugged Donald and our friends, while vowing to do all we could to get help, get them out and get everyone safely back to Ouesso.

We, however, had no idea how we would do so.

Eduardo, David and I walked slowly back through the village, discussing strategy and options. When we were almost to the guesthouse, we heard Matoo's whistle. Quickly turning around, we saw Matoo running toward us. Running a few feet behind him were Donald and Hema.

With great joy, we embraced each other as Donald spoke and David translated.

"The chief officer let them go for the night! They have to go back with us in the morning to see what our punishment is going to be. But they don't have to spend the night in jail!"

Although running away was tempting, it was not an option. The chief officer had our passports, and without them, we could not travel as far as the next region because identification would be required upon entry.

Plus, we would have easily been caught, only to face a greater wrath.

At the guesthouse, we sat and talked until early morning. It seemed that no one wanted to go to sleep. No one wanted to be alone.

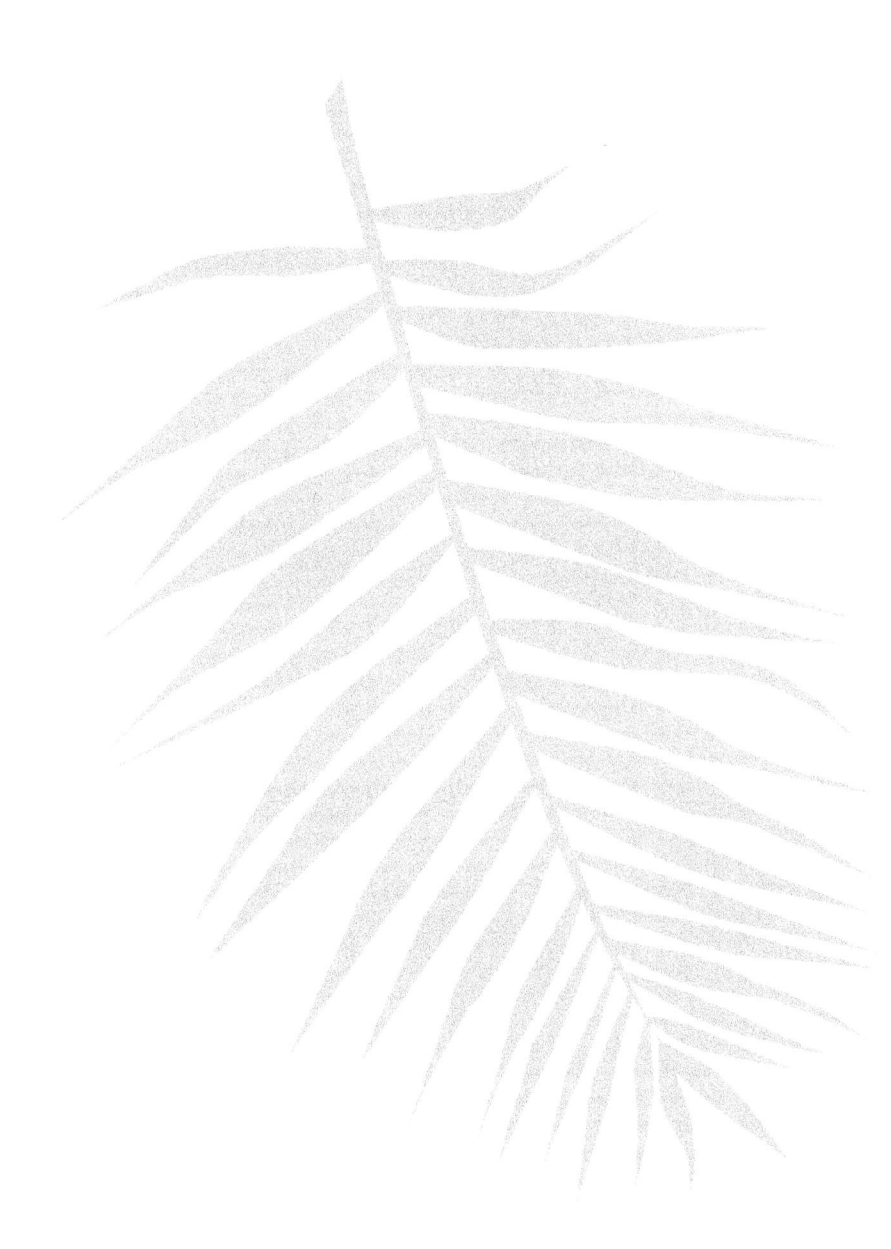

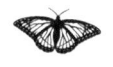
Chapter Twenty-Eight

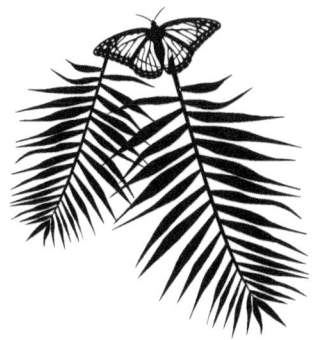

The following morning, we left the guesthouse early and walked back to the police building. As we made our way up the hill, the chief officer leaned across the porch's railing, watching us closely. Reaching the structure, we climbed the three steps and walked toward him, apologizing once again for any misunderstandings or problems we had created.

As the seven of us gathered around the officer, Eduardo, David, Donald and I continued talking while the officer remained silent. Gone were the anger and rage he spewed only hours earlier. With a calmness and even a gentleness, he listened without interrupting.

After several minutes, the officer reached into his dark green military-style jacket and pulled out our passports and Donald's necklace. Then, extending his arm, he handed them to us while speaking for the first time.

"He says that we should not have been on the river after dark . . . that the next time we come to the village, we need to discuss our plans—everything—with him first. That way he knows where—and what—we are doing at all times," David translated from Donald's French.

"Yes," I responded. "We promise. Thank you. We apologize for not knowing better."

"*Merci,*" David and Eduardo chimed in. *"Merci beaucoup!"*

As the officer shook each of our hands, he smiled, and we were allowed to leave.

Minutes after leaving the police quarters, as we walked through the village, a man standing beside a nearby hut whistled and motioned us over. Donald insisted that we head back to the guesthouse while he went to see what the man wanted.

It was then that Donald learned the complete story.

"The man told Donald that he was the one who went to the police and begged them to let us go," David translated.

"Wait . . . I'm not getting this. I can't figure out what Donald is trying to say. Hold on, let me ask him again."

For a few minutes David and Donald spoke in French as Donald elaborated.

"Ohhh," David exclaimed, "Now I understand.

You're not going to believe this.

This guy Donald met just returned from Pokola. The guy was visiting his brother who lives there. His brother told him about the three white people who came to their village. And flew drones and were arrested.

He told how President Sassou Nguesso protected the white people and was upset with the officers who arrested them. And then talked about the two helicopters in the village.

So, last night when this guy heard that white people had been arrested, he thought it had to be the same ones. So, he went to the

Chapter Twenty-Eight

police building and told the story he had heard in Pokola to one of the subordinate officers.

This is wild . . ." David said.

"Donald said that when this guy told the story to the chief officer, he begged the officers not to put us in jail or to harm us because the President was protecting us.

When we were put in the side room with Hema, Matoo and the boat driver . . . that's when this guy was talking to the officers."

"You've got to be kidding!" I said. "What are the chances? Seriously. What are the chances anyone from this tiny village would have traveled to Pokola? And traveled right after our arrest in Pokola? Only to return at a critical time? And then help us?"

"It's unreal," David responded. "If it wasn't for him, we could be in a totally different situation now. We've got to thank him."

"Talk about divine intervention. And protection," I added.

Donald interrupted and began speaking in French to David.

"Ahhh. There's a really good reason we were in so much trouble being on the river after dark. It's a serious crime.

There's a shitload of diamonds in this area. Donald says that you can find them laying on the ground.

With no mining companies, the area is still pristine. Pretty much untouched.

At night though, the diamonds are trafficked in boats down the river. Then sold on the black market.

They thought we were smuggling diamonds. That's why they were so mad."

When David finished the translation, I asked Donald why we had not been told about the smuggling. Adding that we would never have intentionally broken a law.

"He says that we have permits," David relayed. "There are

exceptions to the law and because of our permits, we should have been exempt.

Donald is saying we should never have had a problem. The officer chose to make it a problem."

It was our last day in the village and even though the original plan was to spend several hours with the Baka healer Lakuneta, it was tempting to simply go ahead and leave the village. We were emotionally drained and anxious, fearing that it was only a matter of time before the police confronted us again and charged us with something else. Every minute we remained in the village felt as if we were further testing fate.

But I asked that we take the time.

"We don't have a lot of time left, so let's grab our day packs and camera gear and go to Lakuneta's village. I'd like to spend at least two hours with him. Is that possible? Is that okay?" I asked.

"By my calculations, we need to be on the river in three and a half hours at the very latest in order to make it to Ouesso by dark. Anything later than that, we will have to stay another night in the village. We can't risk being on the river after dark, especially knowing what we do now." Eduardo responded.

"If we spend two hours with Lakuneta," David added, "that'll still give enough time to pack up, transport the gear and load the boat. I'm ready to get back to Ouesso, guys. I'm afraid if we stay another day, there'll be something else they'll arrest us for . . . we may not be so lucky the next time."

Chapter Twenty-Eight

At the guesthouse, we grabbed the cameras and day packs and then made the trip to Lakuneta's village in twenty minutes. Seven minutes faster than on the previous day.

The village was quiet.

In the distance, children ran between huts and women gathered in a small circle. To our left, Lakuneta sat outside the hut he called home, on a short tree stump. Composed of wooden planks stacked horizontally, five feet in height, the rectangular structure housed a single room. Layers of dried grass created a roof, which extended three feet beyond the structure's wooden walls, shading Lakuneta who sat underneath.

Hearing our approach, Lakuneta stood and smiled. When he did, a sense of peace immediately overwhelmed me.

The encounters with the officers resulted in days riddled with apprehension and anxiety. But Lakuneta's smile magically made the angst disappear.

On the day prior, while we traveled the river visiting other villages, Lakuneta and his helper, who was a young man in his thirties, went into the jungle to collect medicine to share with us. Roots, leaves, bark and stems lay on the ground, separated and bound by vines.

After handshakes and greetings, Lakuneta's helper placed several small tree stumps in front of Lakuneta and motioned for us to sit. Lakuneta sat first, followed immediately by his helper. On the ground in between them lay the small heap of plants.

Lakuneta's baggy dark blue pants appeared several sizes too big. Beneath the rolled-up pants' legs—whose fabric still managed to drag the ground—were calloused feet covered in layers of dirt. An oversized yellow-brown shirt missing several buttons swallowed his small frame.

Donald spoke first and David translated.

"Donald is telling Lakuneta about our arrest . . . and the problems we had last night. And this morning. And why we are later than we had planned.

He's apologizing for not being here earlier," David relayed.

While Donald spoke, Lakuneta responded with frequent deep, short groans as if saying 'ahhh' before eventually speaking.

"Lakuneta is saying that he is sorry we had problems. He doesn't want us to worry. Time does not matter."

Donald then turned and nodded to me. A sign that it was time for me to talk.

"Thank you for allowing us to spend time with you, Lakuneta. It is a great honor to be with you," I said. "And thank you for your kindness and understanding. Our journey has had many challenges. Including the arrest last night.

You have been a highlight of our trip in many ways."

With David and Donald translating, the conversation continued.

"He thanks us for coming," David said. "He is very happy we are here. They have never had people like us—outsiders—to come to their village. No one has ever asked how they live . . . or about their medicine.

He is happy to share their medicine because their medicine is good medicine. And he wants to help people. Even those he does not know."

As Lakuneta spoke, several members of the tribe gathered around us, sitting quietly on the ground.

One by one, the vines that held bundles of plants together were

Chapter Twenty-Eight

untied by his helper while Lakuneta talked in depth about the treatments. He told the name of the plant and its use, how it was prepared and administered. He spoke of many remedies including for infections, pain and toothaches.

For inflammation, he scraped the inner layer of a bark, boiled the shavings, and then had the person drink several ounces of the liquid three times a day. For insomnia or difficulty sleeping, he added water to the scrapings of another tree's bark and then placed the drops directly into a person's eyes.

Constantly during the conversation, Lakuneta squinted. His eyes almost closed.

"Lakuneta, may I ask about your eyesight?" I inquired.

He smiled. And gave a lengthy response.

"When he was born, he could not see. He was blind," David translated.

"He says he has not seen things that others have seen.

His father was a great healer and before him, his father's father . . . and before him, his grandfather's father. For as long as anyone can remember. Because his father loved him so deeply, and because he was the first-born male child, he was also taught to be a healer.

Even though he could not see, his father taught him about the medicines of the forest and all that he knew, so that Lakuneta could take his place one day. And help his village too."

As Donald and David translated, I sat in silence.

"His father would take Lakuneta's hands and make him feel the trees . . . the bushes . . . the leaves . . . the roots. He made him smell them so he would know them. Many plants he had him taste," David relayed.

"Now, when Lakuneta goes into the forest, he takes someone with him. When he finds the medicine, he tells his helper, 'Cut from this tree, but not from that one' and 'Take leaves from this plant, but not from that one.'

This is how he helps others."

As I listened to his story and as he described each medicine in the small pile, I realized that I was not only sitting in the presence of a remarkable medicine man . . .

I was in the presence of a most unique gift from God.

After the conversation, Lakuneta's helper placed a handmade stringed instrument on Lakuneta's lap. The triangular-shaped instrument's base was a thin, three-foot-long piece of wood that gently pressed across Lakuneta's stomach. At the wood's midpoint, a narrow six-inch piece of wood protruded outward, toward his knees. On the smaller piece of wood, near its far end, were carved three slight indentions.

Running through each indention was a tightly bound string whose ends were attached to either end of the instrument's larger wooden base. Making forty-five-degree angles to the base.

Lakuneta announced that as a gift he would sing and play for us.

Moving his hands, Lakuneta altered the locations in which his fingers strummed the three strings. While he performed, other members of the tribe clapped and danced.

Lakuneta's father honored his son's birthright and never allowed Lakuneta's blindness to interfere or inhibit his role as the village's healer. According to the members of the village that

Chapter Twenty-Eight

day, no one knew the medicine better—and no one could play the instrument or sing more beautifully than Lakuneta.

Before leaving, I placed an anklet around Lakuneta's right foot. The crafted adornment, which had been made by a friend, Theresa, who was also the Healing Seekers' bookkeeper, had been blessed by several ministers, clergy and spiritual leaders in the U.S. before our departure.

Such an anklet had been given to every healer since our very first expedition.

Tying it securely around his ankle, I placed my hands lightly on top of it and around his ankle. As I did so, I told Lakuneta that the leather woven band was a symbol of our love and prayers for him.

Prayers for his continued health and happiness . . .

For days filled with love and joy . . .

Prayers for his safety . . . and that of his family and village . . .

Until we meet again.

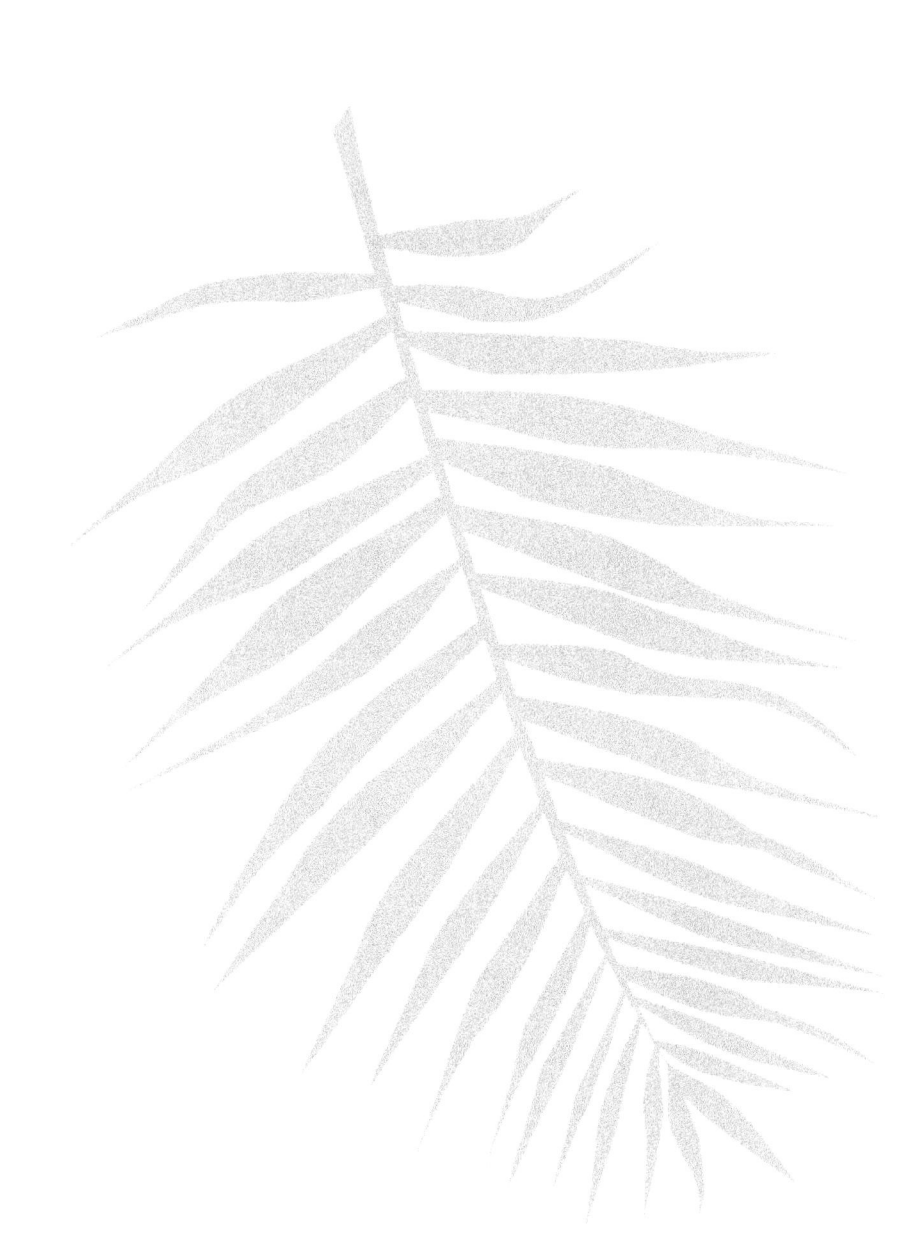

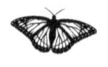
Chapter Twenty-Nine

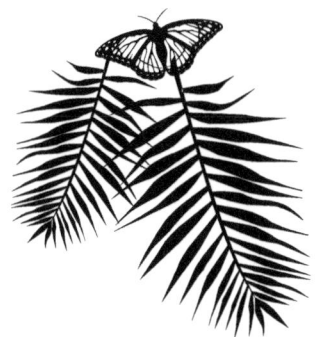

Time was tight, so we hurried back to the guesthouse to pack the final items. Eduardo was first to leave for the boat, accompanying the porters and two young boys Donald had hired to help carry the bags and equipment. A few minutes later, Donald left for the immigration officer's building to document our departure. Following closely behind him, after packing all the remaining items and settling up with the owner of the guesthouse, David and I, too, left for the river.

We had gotten ready in record time. With a little over an hour to spare, we were comfortably ahead of schedule.

As David and I passed through the village, we heard a man yell as if trying to get someone's attention. Looking around, we saw a man waving as he walked toward us. When he got closer, we realized he was the subordinate officer who had interrogated the porters and boat driver in the separate room during our arrest. Smiling, he shook both our hands and spoke in French, which David translated. His demeanor was the complete opposite of what we had experienced earlier at the police quarters. He was so kind that one would have thought we were all close friends.

While we talked, and also apologized again for our actions and for the misunderstanding, he looked beyond us, over our left shoulders and said, *"Le chef veut que vous veniez à lui."*

David translated, "Their village chief wants to see us."

Thirty yards away, a man who looked to be in his seventies stood in front of a hut and raised his hand, as if to say 'here I am.' In front of him, sitting on the ground in a semi-circle, was a group of nine male elders.

With a final handshake and a good-bye to the subordinate officer, we turned and walked in the direction of the chief. Before reaching him, we had to pass by five of the elders who sat on the ground. As we did so, we greeted each of them with *"bonjour."*

But not one of them answered. Not one of them smiled.

There was no warmth or even a hint of kindness. It was completely different from the lighthearted and even joyful officer whom we had just left.

A sinking feeling hit hard in the pit of my stomach. Something wasn't right.

Before we got within an arm's reach of the chief, he turned and started walking away from us, down a narrow grass path toward the jungle. Even without speaking, we knew we were to follow.

With every step, we were led deeper into the woods and farther away from the village. No one on our team knew where we were, and we had no idea where we were going. We had no choice but to follow, for to run would not only be disrespectful, but such an action might imply that we were guilty of something.

The chief walked several feet ahead of me. David, meanwhile, walked only steps behind me so that we could whisper to one another.

"What the hell? Where is he taking us? What have we done? What is he going to do to us?"

Chapter Twenty-Nine

For ten minutes we followed the chief along the overgrown trail through the woods until he led us to an opening under a large tree. Beneath its overhanging limbs were three simple wooden chairs and a small wooden table. The largest chair faced west and was pushed against the table, which seemed to function as a desk. The other two chairs were placed in front of the desk, facing east. As he sat in the chair behind the desk, he motioned for us to sit in the other two.

Just as he was beginning to talk, Donald came running through the woods. Thankfully, someone in the village had gone to him and told him where we were being taken. Out of breath, he spoke in short sentences to the village chief, tapping lightly on his wristwatch, explaining our need to get on the river quickly.

The chief gave little attention to Donald's pleas, and instead, directed his full attention to David and me as he spoke. With his efforts thwarted and without any power, Donald stood to our right and translated the chief's words to French.

David then leaned closer to me and translated the words to English: "The chief wants us to know that he has greater power than the police. The next time we visit, we are to come to him first."

I asked David and Donald to translate as I apologized for not knowing better and that we intended no disrespect. It was an honor to meet him— a man of such power. We promised that on all future trips, we would come to him first.

David translated my words and added that we would look forward to spending time with him and hearing more about his life.

Donald, in the meantime, fidgeted as he stared at his watch. Sighing heavily, he tried once more to interrupt the chief and explain that we needed to leave.

The chief, however, insisted that we remain until he was finished.

As the chief reiterated his previous points and his words were translated, David and I responded that we understood. Satisfied, the chief announced that we could leave.

Before leaving, I asked if I might take a quick photo with him. To which, he proudly accepted. After taking several photos, he walked a few feet to a nearby tree and picked two beautiful limes from its branches and placed them in my hands. Smiling, he asked that another photo be taken.

The chief had heard that there were three of us. And insisted on also meeting Eduardo, who was waiting by the boat with the others. Although Donald tried to quicken our pace, the chief leisurely strolled while demanding that Donald slow down and translate so that he could have more of a conversation with David and me.

The chief inquired, "Where in the United States do you live? What do you do there? How long did it take you to get to Congo? Are you married? Why not? Do you have children? Why not?"

When we were in sight of our teammates at the river, one of the porters ran to Donald and, in a panic, told him that the immigration officer had come to the river looking for him. The officer demanded to speak further—he was not approving our departure. We were not allowed to leave.

Infuriated, Donald took off and ran toward the immigration officer's building, located a half mile away.

"What's going on?" David and I asked Eduardo and the porters. "Donald has already cleared the departure with the immigration officer. He stamped our paperwork. What's the problem?"

"Guys, we have no idea," Eduardo replied. "He was really mad! And kept pointing to the boat—forbidding us to leave."

"You've got to be kidding me. Seriously?" I quipped.

"Don't worry I'm sure Donald will take care of it." David added.

Chapter Twenty-Nine

"Hmmm . . . Do you think we should go to the office and make sure he is okay?"

"Let's give him twenty minutes," Eduardo said. "If we aren't on the river by then, we're going to have to stay another night anyway."

"This is unreal!" David added. "What if they won't let us leave?"

While Eduardo, Matoo and I sat on an old log and nervously waited, David stood impatiently a few feet away. With each passing minute, our hopes of leaving the village and reaching Ouesso that day began to fade. There was a limited amount of daylight to make the journey, and if we did not leave soon, we would find ourselves on the river in the dark. Potentially setting us up for yet another arrest.

Because of the meeting with the village chief, we were dangerously close to being behind schedule. Finally, with only five minutes to spare, our boat driver spotted Donald running full stride in the distance down the dirt road. Raising high his right arm and moving it in a big circle as if he had a lasso, Donald pointed at us as if to say, 'let's go.'

At his gestures, the boat driver rushed to the back of the dugout, pulled the cord and started the motor. After quickly saying good-bye to the village chief and giving him a hug, I boarded the boat after the others. Donald, in the meantime, appeared a couple of feet behind me, shoving the boat further into the water before jumping inside with the rest of us.

Motoring away, we turned around and stared at the departure point, fearing that one of the officers would suddenly appear and summon us to return. The further away we traveled, however, the more relaxed we became. When the clearing along the river bank was no longer in sight, I sighed heavily and smiled.

David yelled, "We made it!"

Laughing, I leaned back and gave him a high five. "Woohoo!" I exclaimed.

"That was close," Eduardo responded. "Just a few more minutes and we would have had to stay another night."

Even though the river might bring other issues and problems, none of those problems would be the constant apprehension and dread of the officers from the village. And that thought alone seemed to instantly free us from the emotional and psychological bondage in which we had been imprisoned since our arrival.

The water was soothing as it rippled against the boat. I gazed far into the distance, knowing that somewhere out there was Ouesso.

And somewhere out there was our friend, Denise.

Chapter Thirty

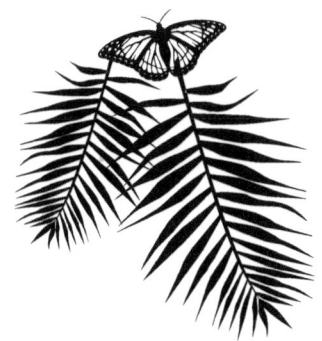

Because it was dry season, the river's water was low. The boat driver, therefore, had to go back and forth across the width of the river, from the banks of the Congo to the banks of Cameroon and back again in order to follow the deeper water within the main current. Unfortunately, the water in the main current often became shallow as well, and due to the great deal of weight in our boat, on several occasions, we hit the bottom of the river.

Five times the boat became stranded on sandbars. Five times we had to push and pull and wiggle the boat out of its entrapments.

The groundings, as well as the weavings back and forth across the river, added time we had not anticipated. When the sun began its descent behind the trees, we were still a little over five kilometers away from Ouesso. It was a situation I had prayed we would not face.

I began to search the banks of the river for possible sites to pitch camp, but no matter how hard I looked, there were no natural openings in the thick foliage. Pitching camp on unknown territory and on land that belonged to an unknown tribe could be catastrophic. And yet, remaining on the river after dark had its own consequences.

I turned and looked at Donald who sat in the back of the boat, directly in front of the boat driver. The outboard motor and the splashing water made it impossible to yell loud enough for him to hear me, so I pointed to my wrist as if I had a watch and gave a thumbs up and then a thumbs down, nonverbally asking if our timing was still good. Although he nodded his head yes, his facial expression said otherwise. He then turned and motioned for the driver to hurry.

The sun eventually disappeared completely behind the trees until its glow of red, orange and yellow turned various shades of gray. And then a dark gray.

Our chances of arriving to Ouesso in time were slim, but Donald insisted it was possible. Even though the loss of light warranted our head lamps, we refrained from turning them on because doing so would admit that we were on the river after dark.

There was only a sliver of light remaining on the horizon when the entry point to Ouesso came within sight. A single light along the edge of the river shown brightly and the driver sped directly toward it. According to Eduardo, as we pulled alongside the wooden platform underneath the light, we had six minutes to spare.

Bags were quickly unloaded from the boat and tossed onto the wobbly platform that rocked with the water. Turning on our head lamps, we picked up the bags and carried them up the hill, where immigration officers were waiting for us.

They laughed as one of the officers pointed to his watch and said, "Presque en retard," which meant 'almost late.'

Pulling out our passports, we handed them to the two officers who opened and inspected each one. They then asked where we had been and where we were going before collecting entry fees for each of us. It was a normal process and a requirement for anyone entering the city.

Chapter Thirty

As Donald and I cleared the paperwork with the immigration officers, Eduardo and David hired a local man to drive us into town. Saying good-bye to our boat driver, and goodnight to Donald, who lived nearby, we loaded the vehicle and headed to Denise's restaurant.

The restaurant was located along a dead-end dirt road, wide enough for only one vehicle. The driver stopped a few feet from the eight-foot-high wooden gates that blocked the view of the small establishment behind.

After settling up with the driver, we grabbed our bags and pushed open the gates. Forty feet away, Denise sat at a table. Seeing her, we dropped the bags and rushed to her. At the same time, she quickly stood and yelled, "Ahhh!"

It was the first time in weeks that we felt protected . . . and safe. It was the first time in weeks that we knew everything was going to be okay. Simply being in her presence—our Congolese mother— we knew that there was nothing else to fear . . . and nothing further about which to worry.

As she embraced each of us, tears formed in my eyes.

And in David's.

And in Eduardo's.

For hours we sat, eating and drinking while recounting the details of the trek. We told of the helicopters and the bees, ants and lack of water. We described the fear of being lost and our despair,

And the Silent Spoke

thinking that we would never see our family and friends again.

We spoke of the incidents with the police and being on the river after dark—and how the man in the village, who had just returned from Pokola, went to the officers when we were arrested and begged them not to harm us. We shared the stories of the Baka medicine and the happy songs that Lakuneta had played and sang for us, and then recounted the ordeals of the river trip to Ouesso with the boat getting stuck multiple times and our concern about being arrested again for being on the river after dark.

While we sat and talked, Denise insisted that we needed to eat and eat, stating that we had lost much weight and were not healthy. As the food continued to appear on our table, I was struck with a profound thought: Not once during the entire trip had Eduardo, David and I been left alone. No matter the challenges, struggles, 'failures,' and fears, there had been many others—many angels—supporting, protecting, and walking with us.

They were angels in the forms of restaurant owners and Ambassadors, Colonels and Presidents, managers of guesthouses, porters, trackers, villagers, translators and healers. And I was certain that there were many more who remained unknown and unseen.

The angels made our path easier and the hurdles surmountable. They strengthened our faith and drove further our devotion. They arrived at the perfect times and often during the darkest hours . . . holding our hands and encouraging us when we needed it most.

Had it not been for Denise in particular, we would have likely continued to believe the lies of the logistics team and succumb to their threats, resulting in a failed expedition that would have prevented us from seeing the true beauty of the Congo and the Congolese people. It would have also most likely led to the demise of Healing Seekers.

Chapter Thirty

We talked well into the night. And eventually retired to sleep in the extra rooms that Denise owned and managed.

It was the best night's sleep any of us had had in weeks.

As we hugged Denise the following morning for the last time, each of us fought through heightened emotions and tears. As did she.

Mumbling, I stuttered, "Thank you. For everything."

There was so much more I wanted to say, but my emotions took over, and even the words 'I love you' became mere utterances of incomprehensible sounds.

Somehow, though, it was okay.

Somehow . . . I knew that she had heard all that my heart longed to say.

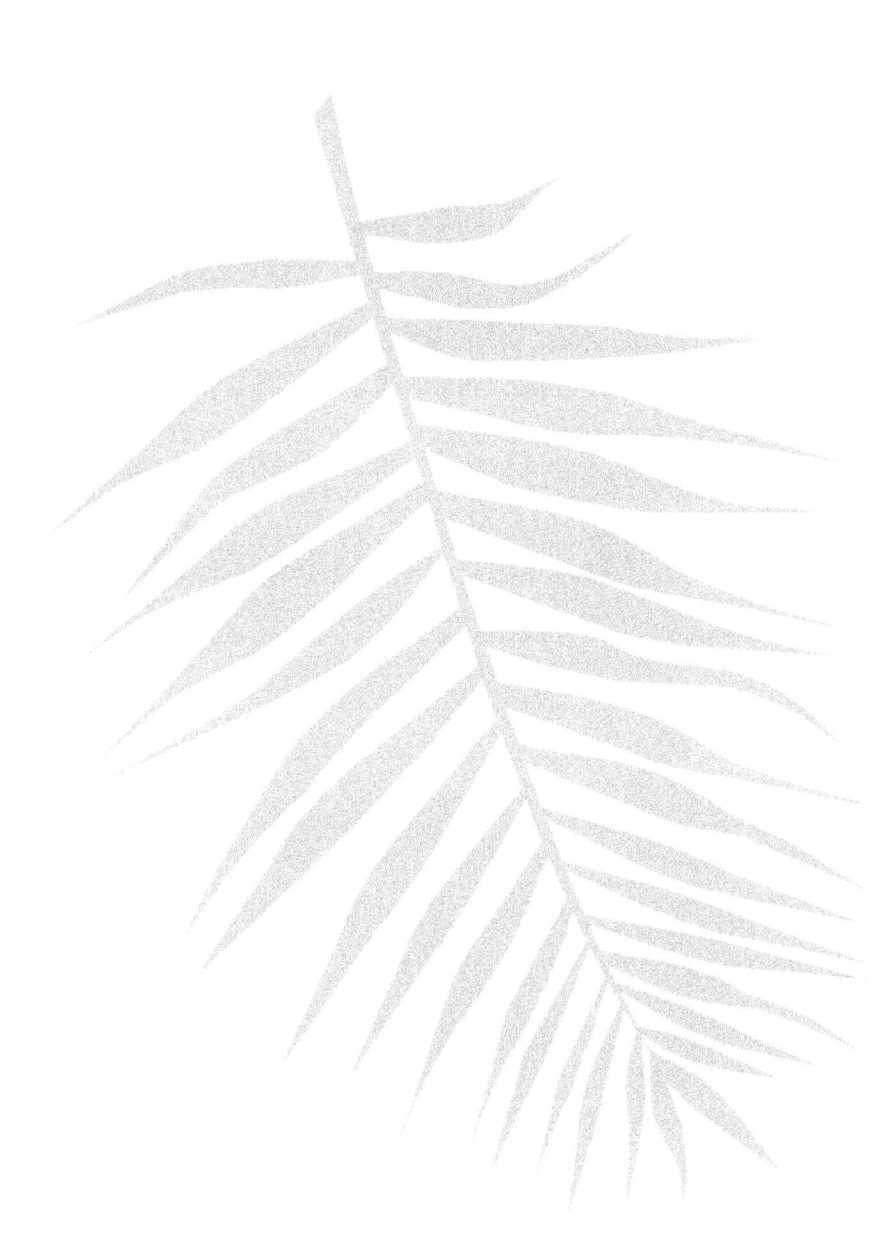

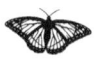
Chapter Thirty-One

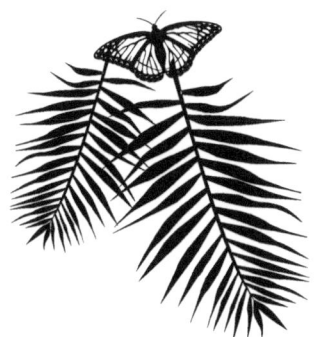

Love transcends both the unspoken and spoken word. It is uninhibited by time, space or dimension. Distance or death. Love never fails.

Even when life refuses to grant a moment to say good-bye . . . or an opportunity to say I love you . . . one more time.

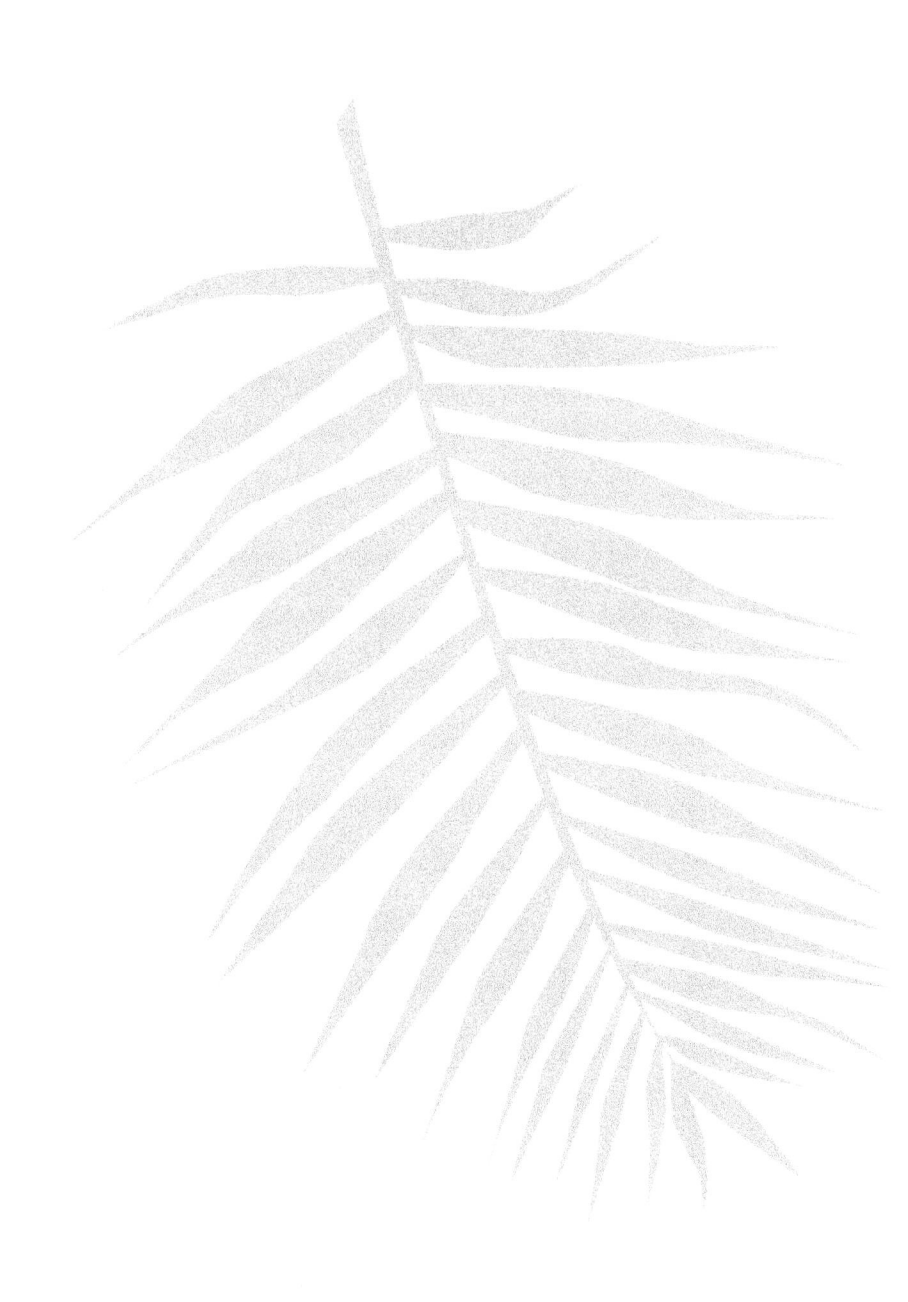

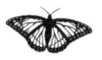
Chapter Thirty-Two

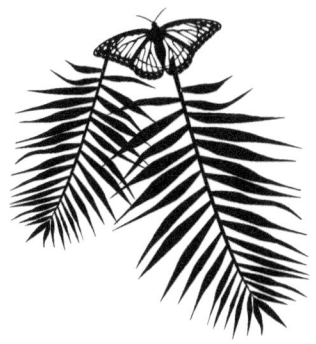

She turned to look at her nieces and nephews, but when she did, her vision blurred and a strange sensation took hold of her body. As if she were dreaming and hallucinating at the same time—people suddenly appeared before her: her partner and her parents, her grandparents, aunts and uncles—and many other loved ones who had long departed the earthly world. Among them were also Johamad and Kupsey, Malahe and Denise, and even the chief from Jimson's village.

Their presence brought an indescribable joy, making even the cells in her body seem to dance. She felt light and free, protected and uninhibited.

As they drew closer to her, she drew closer to them. And much like an infant who is tenderly cradled in its mother's arms, she surrendered completely to the love that enveloped her—a love so strong, it brought tears to her eyes.

She had never had such peace.

With a smile, she looked at her partner and parents, and took a long, deep breath and slowly exhaled.

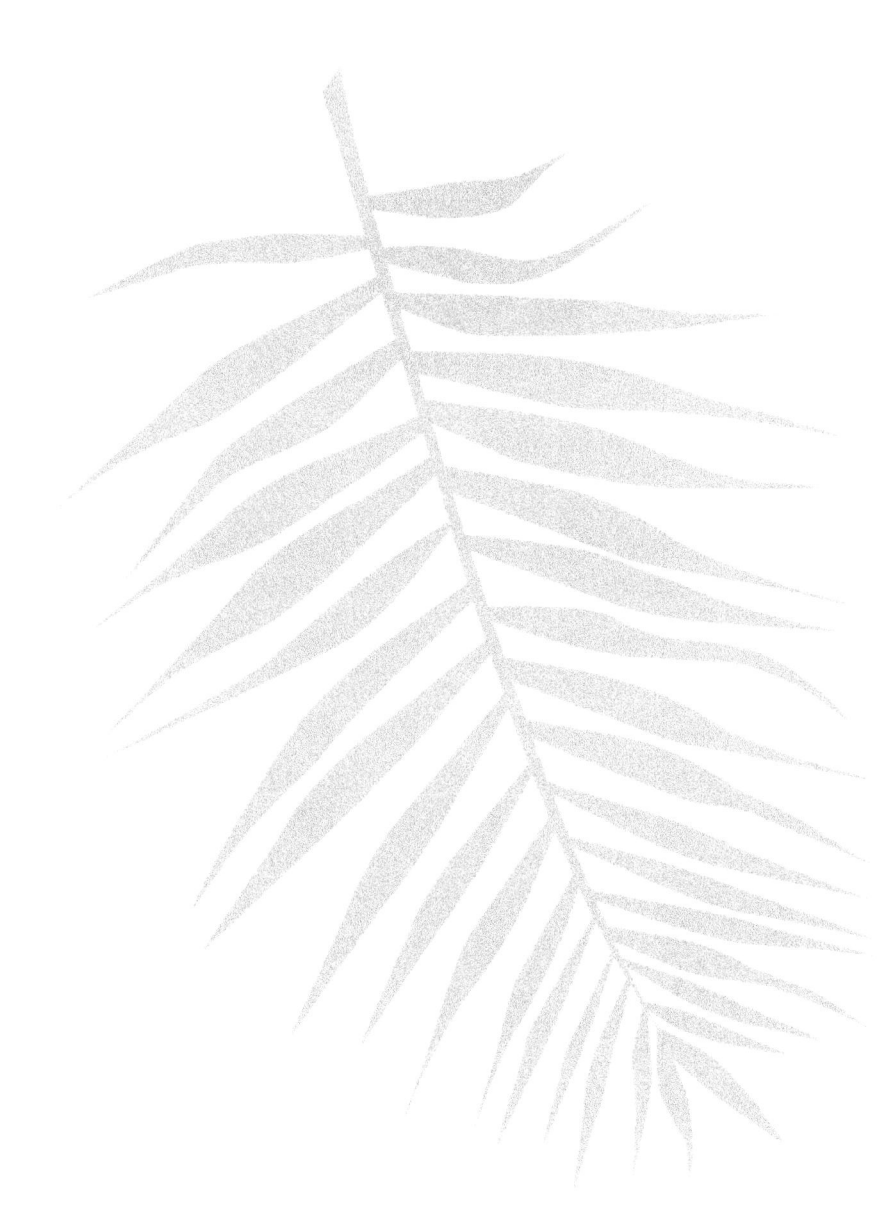

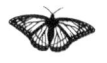
Chapter Thirty-Three

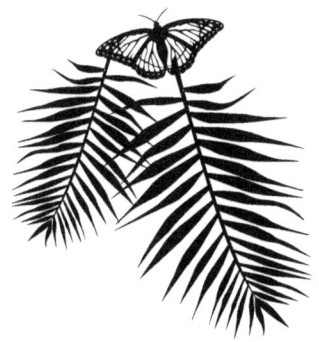

A s she took the deep breath, the nieces and nephews watched in silence as she slowly exhaled.
The breath she drew would turn out to be her last.
And with it, she would be the first to say good-bye.

The kids had surrounded her for three days. But during those days, she had never uttered a word, never opened her eyes.

It had only been a few hours before they arrived at the airport that Dominga had discovered her lying unresponsive in her bed at home. Trails of dried tears were streaked across her cheeks, while pieces of broken mirror lay scattered upon the hardwood floor beneath her hand, which dangled off the side of the bed.

A massive stroke. The severity of which was so extreme that she never regained consciousness. During the three days, the nieces and nephews watched over her like ever-faithful guardians. Surrounding her bed in the small hospital room, they watched her breaths become more and more labored as she weakened by the hour.

She seemed to be at peace—and at times, even appearing to smile.

But there were other times when she tensed and became agitated, and it was during those moments that they spoke softly to her and gently held her hand. And when her hands felt cold, they placed warm blankets over her, tucking the edges snugly around her.

Doctors, nurses and staff came in and out of the room constantly, keeping her comfortable, monitoring medications and often entering the room to silence the obnoxious beeps of the IVs and equipment. Much like the beeping sounds made when trucks back up, or the sounds of a monotonous ring tones, the noises frequently startled and irritated her. The constant muffled sounds of the hospital's intercom system also added to her unease.

In the mornings, the room smelled of Moravian sugar cake and the kids' coffees, teas and lattes. At other times, scents stemmed from the meals and snacks that had so carefully been planned and prepared. Twice, Dominga delivered outside food, which brought yet another plethora of aromas—sandwiches, burgers and fries from Cafe Arthur's and North Carolina barbecue with hushpuppies and slaw.

As they sat only inches away from her, the nieces and nephews reminisced about their childhoods and their later years in life, while also recalling many of the stories they had heard about their aunt and her expeditions.

As they chatted, they had many questions. Details they longed to hear, including her innermost feelings. The questions, however, remained unanswered, as her voice remained silent and her body, almost motionless.

The days had passed quickly, and there was a deep sadness for the loss. And a greater one for not knowing the purpose for which they had been summoned.

Little did they know, however, that it had been during those three days

Chapter Thirty-Three

that she had shared all the things left unsaid . . . and communicated all the things she had longed to say. She had showered them with love while her soul had soared . . . and her heart had burst with joy.

And it was from that realm, not so far away,
Where Love alone is known,
That while they gathered one last time,
Messages were imprinted upon their hearts—and minds.

Life is precious, every being a gift,
Each with value, purpose—many reasons to exist.
On mountains, valleys and in the seas,
Within the jungles of plants and trees,
To thrive, and yet provide—the world its many needs.

Life will whither, bodies cease to breathe,
So make paramount your mission, and refuse to leave
A world without kindness, empathy . . . good deeds.
And, especially, your love within it weaved.

Along the journey upon this Earth,
Through times of discovery and re-birth,
Listen often during the days and weeks.

For from the stillness will emerge . . .
The faint whisperings of the words . . .
That God—and All the silent—speak.

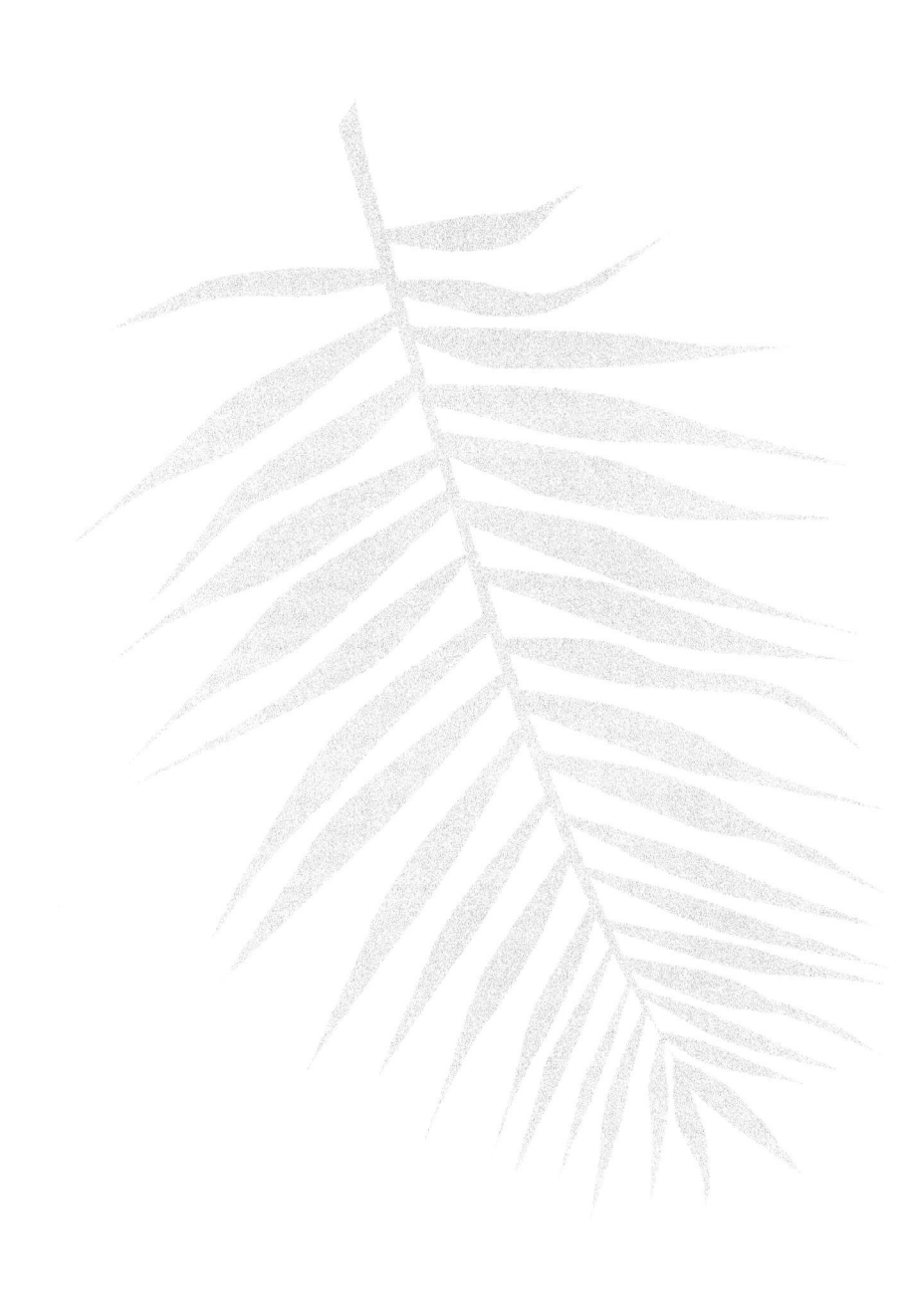

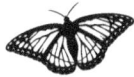

About the Author

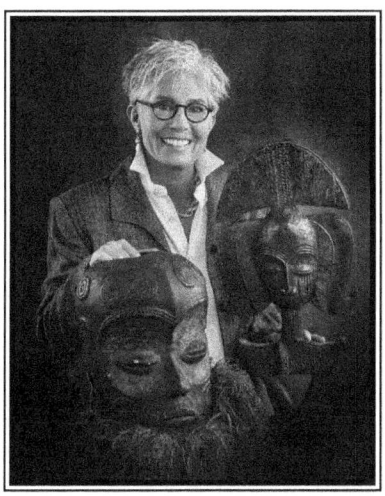

A my Greeson, graduate of UNC-Chapel Hill Eshelman School of Pharmacy and member of the Pharmacy School's Alumni Board of Directors, has traveled extensively to study indigenous healing methods and plant-based medicine. She has led multiple treks to remote, isolated regions of the planet, including to the Amazon, Madagascar, Papua New Guinea and the Republic of the Congo, to bring awareness of indigenous cultures and their environments, and to further research in the pursuit of novel medical treatments.

Amy is the founder of Healing Seekers, a non-profit which creates educational materials, and is co-founder of Natural Discoveries, Inc., a natural products discovery research company. She lives in High Point,

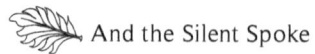 And the Silent Spoke

North Carolina, with her significant other and their dog, Congo. In her free time, she enjoys photography and collecting art, especially within the regions she has explored.

www.ingramcontent.com/pod-product-compliance
Lightning Source LLC
Chambersburg PA
CBHW051556010526
44118CB00023B/2731